Marti,

Enjoy working with you!

Best of luck/success.

Tom Miller

The Jossey-Bass/AHA Press Series translates the latest ideas on health care management into practical and actionable terms. Together, Jossey-Bass and the American Hospital Association offer these essential resources for the health care leaders of today and tomorrow.

◆ ◆

Health Care Strategy
for Uncertain Times

Marian C. Jennings, Editor

· ·

Health Care Strategy for Uncertain Times

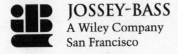
JOSSEY-BASS
A Wiley Company
San Francisco

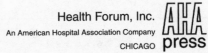
Health Forum, Inc.
An American Hospital Association Company
CHICAGO press

Library of Congress Cataloging-in-Publication Data
Health care strategy for uncertain times / Marian C. Jennings, editor.
    p. ; cm. — (Jossey-Bass/AHA Press series)
    Includes bibliographical references and index.
    ISBN 0-7879-5505-1 (hc : alk. paper)
    1. Health services administration. 2. Strategic planning. 3. Health planning. 4. Health facilities—Planning. I. Jennings, Marian C. II. Series.
    [DNLM: 1. Health Services Administration. 2. Financial Management. 3. Health Care Sector—trends. 4. Health Planning—organization & administration. W 84.1 H43717 2000]
RA971 .H3865 2000
362.1'068—dc21
                                                                    00-033073

FIRST EDITION
HB Printing 10 9 8 7 6 5 4 3 2 1

Contents

. . . .

List of Figures and Tables

. . . .

Chapter Four

Chapter Five

Chapter Six

Chapter Seven

Chapter Eight

Chapter 9

Acknowledgments

This book could not have been written without the insight and assistance of many people. I would like first to thank our clients, many of whom have worked with our firm for years and from whom we continue to learn so much about the practical application of planning theory. Second, I would like to acknowledge the contributions of our entire consulting staff, all of whom participated in conceptualizing, debating about, and actually writing the book. Finally, I would like to thank two individuals without whose efforts this book would not exist: Jennifer Swartz Turfle, for guiding this manuscript through its numerous draft stages with great care; and Edwin P. Ewing Jr., M.D., for providing his insight and clarity of expression.

MARIAN C. JENNINGS
Editor

Introduction

. . . .

The health care industry is in the midst of a fundamental, often painful, restructuring. Major health care systems and hospitals that long have enjoyed success and dominance no longer assume that their future is ensured. Community hospitals worry about their ability to remain independent while continuing to pursue their mission of service to all those in need. Rural hospitals, often serving an older and sicker population, worry about their ability to survive as a needed community resource. Physicians no longer hold the social or economic status that they enjoyed as recently as a decade ago. As for managed care plans, having obtained in the mid-1990s easy, first-generation discounts and utilization reductions, they now struggle to control costs to maintain their own financial viability. All the players—providers, physicians, and insurers alike—stand on the threshold of biotechnology and information technology advances that will transform what is meant by health, health care, health care delivery, and health care financing.

The rapidly changing industry structures require a changed strategic planning approach, as well. Those involved in strategic planning today must recognize that the future of health care in the United States has never been more uncertain. All participants face an increasingly volatile health care market characterized by tremendous financial pressures. This uncertainty can have a debilitating impact on those responsible for strategic planning. Although strategic planning is even more important during times of uncertainty, many feel that it is expendable because no one knows what the future holds. The great uncertainties of the market threaten the risk-averse cultures of many not-for-profit health care organizations. New strategic planning methods must acknowledge and address head on the conflicts between the risks of the environment and the risk-averse cultures of the organizations.

Traditional strategic planning processes often focused on developing broad-based consensus for organizational direction. The planning process often occurred biannually and took many months, not weeks, to accomplish, since there was little sense that the market was moving at a rate that required rapid response. Health care strategy in the twenty-first century requires a faster, continual process— one that transforms the organization, that is led by executive management, that is able to move forward without complete consensus, and that explicitly recognizes both the risks of the marketplace and the fact that not all strategies will be successful, no matter how well conceived. Finally, and perhaps most important, strategy formulation in the future will require an organizational culture that is open to change, willing to learn from its mistakes, and adaptable to a changing environment with emerging and sometimes contradictory rules.

The purpose of this book is to provide health care leaders with the tools to reconceptualize and carry out strategic decision making in a new and unfamiliar environment. The book offers a practical approach based upon our hands-on experience. It presents examples of the tools, techniques, and processes we advocate. We describe three specific techniques, developed in the corporate world, that have been tailored to the unique aspects of the health care industry: scenario planning, decision analysis, and game-theory approaches. In addition, given our bias that strategic planning is ultimately a resource-allocation process, we include guidelines for integrating strategic and financial planning and describe methods for estimating and reducing the financial risks of plan implementation.

We describe facilitation techniques that we have found useful in helping organizations to accept the reality of uncertainty while developing solid strategic direction. Described in the book are new approaches to defining the roles of planning constituents, developing planning assumptions about the future that recognize the uncertainties of the market, developing clear statements of strategic intent in the context of corporate culture, reducing organizational risks by specifying expected outcomes and using metrics, and enhancing organizational readiness to learn and adapt.

The book is organized into ten chapters, around a five-phase strategic planning cycle. Each chapter concludes with a short list of "lessons learned" that reflect our experience in working with health care organizations across the country.

The first three chapters focus on creating understanding in your organization of the nature of risk and uncertainty and establishing an objective, shared understanding of your organization's current competitive positioning. Specifically, Chapter One discusses the differences between risk and uncertainty and presents a framework for understanding the types of uncertainty faced by health care organizations, as well as their root causes. Chapter Two reviews the history of strategic planning efforts in health care and describes the approaches outlined in the remainder of the book, including who should be involved in the process at various points. Chapter Three focuses on the environmental assessment, a critical though often overlooked (or even maligned) component of the strategic direction-setting process. This chapter features a practical approach to ensuring that the environmental assessment is structured to add value to the planning process.

In our experience, one of the most critical steps in the planning process is establishing agreed-upon assumptions about the future environment in which the system or hospital will operate, and what the organization must do well to succeed in that environment. Chapter Four explores the process of developing such planning assumptions, while accepting that the future is not fully knowable and, therefore, planning assumptions cannot describe a single future environment with certainty. The art of planning requires leaders to articulate assumptions about the future that serve as a bridge between the environmental assessment and strategic intent, while realizing that not all assumptions have the same likelihood of occurring.

In some ways, Chapters Five and Six are the heart of this book. That is, they focus on specific approaches to dealing with the uncertainties that health care organizations face and to defining a clear strategic intent—or core ideology, vision, and goals—to move the organization forward in a financially viable manner. Chapter Five reviews three of the classic analytical tools used in the corporate world to address uncertainty. Practical approaches are presented for using these techniques in health care organizations. Chapter Six discusses formulating an organization's strategic intent, including key success factors associated with different types of intent.

Chapters Seven and Eight focus on strategy development and approaches to reducing or managing the risks associated with strategy implementation. Specifically, Chapter Seven discusses the use of clear metrics or measures of success both to help an organization articulate exactly how it wants to be positioned (assuming successful implementation of its strategies) and to help it refocus those strategies that are not accomplishing their objectives. Chapter Eight addresses strategic financial planning in an era of uncertainty; specifically, how financial capability should be allocated to facilitate strategic intent in an era of increasingly limited resources and greater financial risks.

Chapter Nine identifies approaches to help ensure success in the critical implementation phase and identifies the need for compatibility between strategic intent and an organization's culture. The chapter offers guidance for the executive team in managing the human side of the change process.

Finally, Chapter Ten features a brief summary of the aspects of traditional planning that are still appropriate in the new planning era, identifies aspects that should be changed or augmented, and ends with a set of learnings from our experience.

Because this book explores new approaches to strategy formulation in an increasingly uncertain environment, you will be introduced to several new terms, as well as reacquainted with some that are commonly used. Following the final chapter is a Glossary, to familiarize you with these terms.

Our hope in writing this book is that the approach we outline resonates with board members, chief executive officers, vice presidents or directors of strategic planning, chief financial officers, and others involved in the strategic planning process. We hope that you gain insight into the art and the science of strategic planning. We also hope that you see your own organization reflected in some of our examples and that you will have the courage to challenge conventional thinking. Finally, we hope that this book leaves you with at least one "A-ha!" experience.

The Editor and Contributors

Marian C. Jennings, editor, is the president of Jennings Ryan & Kolb. She has worked in the health care industry for twenty-five years. Her first four years were spent in a line management function and the last twenty-one as a health care consultant. Her broad range of experience includes strategic, financial, affiliation, and managed care planning engagements.

Jennings is a frequent speaker and author on the topics of health system integration, physician development strategies, general strategic planning, managed care positioning, and finance. She has presented programs for the American Hospital Association, the Catholic Health Association, the American Medical Association, the Governance Institute, the American College of Healthcare Executives, and the Healthcare Financial Management Association. She was the 1991 recipient of the Corning Award, presented annually by the AHA's Society for Healthcare Planning and Marketing to an individual who has made an outstanding contribution at the national level to the field of health care planning and marketing.

Jennings holds an M.B.A. degree from Harvard University. Prior to cofounding Jennings Ryan & Kolb in 1985, she served as the senior vice president of the Consulting Division of Amherst Associates.

Elizabeth S. Bashore is a consultant of Jennings Ryan & Kolb, in the Jacksonville, Florida, office. She has worked in health care since

1992 and for Jennings Ryan & Kolb since 1999. She holds a master of health care administration degree from the Medical College of Virginia.

Judith E. Belt is a vice president of Jennings Ryan & Kolb and executive-in-charge of the Atlanta office. She has worked in health care since 1981 and for Jennings Ryan & Kolb since 1997. She holds an M.B.A. from the Fuqua School of Business, Duke University.

Tracey L. Camp is a consulting associate of Jennings Ryan & Kolb in the Chicago office. She has worked in health care since 1985 and for Jennings Ryan & Kolb since 1987. She holds a B.A. from Northwestern University.

Erin P. Carr is a manager with TriBrook American Express Tax and Business Services in the Tampa office. She has worked in health care since 1993 and was previously a consultant with Jennings Ryan & Kolb in the Atlanta office. She holds an M.B.A. from Georgia State University.

Cathy Sullivan Clark is a vice president of Jennings Ryan & Kolb and executive-in-charge of the West Springfield, Massachusetts, office. She has worked in health care since 1981 and for Jennings Ryan & Kolb since 1986. She holds a master of management degree from the J. L. Kellogg Graduate School of Management, Northwestern University.

Scott B. Clay is a consultant of Jennings Ryan & Kolb in the Atlanta office. He has worked in health care since 1988 and for Jennings Ryan & Kolb since 1992. He holds an M.B.A. from Emory University.

Ryan S. Gish is a consultant of Jennings Ryan & Kolb in the Chicago office. He has worked in health care since 1995 and for

Jennings Ryan & Kolb since 1997. He holds an M.B.A. from the John M. Olin School of Business, Washington University.

Kathleen Rausch Henchey is a consultant of Jennings Ryan & Kolb in the West Springfield, Massachusetts, office. She has worked in health care since 1985 and for Jennings Ryan & Kolb since 1999. She holds an M.B.A. from the Isenberg School of Management, University of Massachusetts.

Judith L. Horowitz is a vice president of Jennings Ryan & Kolb in the Atlanta office. She has worked in health care consulting since 1982 and for Jennings Ryan & Kolb since 1985. She holds an M.B.A. from Vanderbilt University.

Margo Kelly is a vice president of Jennings Ryan & Kolb in the Jacksonville office. She has worked in health care since 1979 and for Jennings Ryan & Kolb since 1987. She holds M.B.A. and master of hospital administration degrees from Tulane University.

Dennis V. Kennedy is a consultant of Jennings Ryan & Kolb in the West Springfield, Massachusetts, office. He has worked in health care and for Jennings Ryan & Kolb since 1997. He holds a master of science degree in industrial administration from Carnegie Mellon University.

Deborah S. Kolb is an executive vice president of Jennings Ryan & Kolb in the Atlanta office. She has worked in health care since 1979 and for Jennings Ryan & Kolb since 1985. She earned her M.B.A. and Ph.D. at the University of North Carolina at Chapel Hill.

Susanna E. Krentz is a vice president of Jennings Ryan & Kolb and executive-in-charge of the Chicago office. She has worked in health care since 1980 and for Jennings Ryan & Kolb since 1985. She holds an M.B.A. from the University of Chicago.

Thomas R. Miller is a vice president of Jennings Ryan & Kolb in the Chicago office. He has worked in health care since 1981 and for Jennings Ryan & Kolb since 1987. He holds an M.B.A. from the William E. Simon Graduate School of Business Administration, University of Rochester.

J. Bruce Ryan is an executive vice president of Jennings Ryan & Kolb in the Atlanta office. He has worked in health care since 1976 and was a founding partner of Jennings Ryan & Kolb in 1985. He has an M.A. in economics from the University of Washington and an M.S. in finance from the University of Massachusetts.

Carrie S. Stahl is a consultant of Jennings Ryan & Kolb in the Chicago office. She has worked in health care since 1991 and for Jennings Ryan & Kolb since 1999. She holds a master of management degree from the J. L. Kellogg Graduate School of Management, Northwestern University.

J. Edward Witek was a vice president with Jennings Ryan & Kolb, working in the Atlanta office for ten years. He has worked in health care since 1982. He holds a master of health care administration degree from the Medical College of Virginia and an M.B.A. from the University of Hawaii.

Janet S. Young is a consultant of Jennings Ryan & Kolb in the Atlanta office. She has worked in health care since 1994 and for Jennings Ryan & Kolb since 1999. She holds M.B.A. and M.S. (in health administration) degrees from the University of Alabama at Birmingham.

Health Care Strategy
for Uncertain Times

Understanding Risk and Uncertainty

Margo Kelly and Dennis V. Kennedy

Is your market in turmoil? Are the physician or hospital systems that once seemed invincible currently disbanding, divesting, or rethinking their core **strategies**? Do you hear board members or physician leaders lamenting the lost stability of the health care environment of even five years ago? If so, you are not alone. This chapter explores the new reality of health care: that uncertainty is here and will not go away.

To show how uncertainty affects health care organizations, this chapter develops a framework for understanding and characterizing risk and uncertainty. We then discuss how an organization can manage risk through its planning and implementation approaches.

The Reality of Uncertainty

Most health care professionals, whether board members, managers, or physicians, generally would say that the environment they face today is much more uncertain than it was even five years ago. Why? Because, as indicated in Table 1.1, many past predictions have not been realized. Which so-called experts would have predicted that, today, tuberculosis once again is widespread? That capitation is not? That single-signature contracting is not valuable? And that physician practice management companies (PPMs) have been so weakened?

Table 1.1. Past Predictions in Health Care.

Year	Experts Agree That . . .	Instead, Current Reality
1960	Worldwide, TB is controlled.	Drug-resistant strains reappeared in the late 1980s, and TB is currently the world's biggest infectious killer (Moore, 1999a).
1993	Capitation is the payment form of the future.	Only one-third of doctors have any capitated contracts, which account for less than 25 percent of doctors' revenues (Peters, 1999).
1993	Federal health care reform has failed.	Market reforms produced many of the proposed changes (Toner, 1999).
1994	Large hospital systems will have greater negotiating clout with payers.	In many markets, managed care organizations still contract on a hospital-by-hospital basis, regardless of system membership ("Chicago's Northwestern . . . ," 1999).
1997	Physician practice management companies are good investments.	In the first three quarters of 1998, the market capitalization of PPMs plunged from $12.6 billion to $4.4 billion (Hudson, Haugh, and Serb, 1999).

Despite the hopes of many, uncertainty in health care is likely to increase. Figure 1.1 presents but a few of the many major sources of future uncertainty in the industry. Certain sources, such as potential Medicare reform or payer initiatives, directly affect an organization's bottom line. Other sources of uncertainty, such as the timing and extent of medical advances, hint at a profound affect on health care delivery. Every system with a cancer center, faced with the capital costs associated with upgrading imaging and radiation

Figure 1.1. Examples of Future Uncertainties.

Medicare reform

Payments to hospitals were cut $71 billion in 1999 ("A Comprehensive Review . . . ," 1999), with an additional $39 billion in cuts proposed in 1999 ("Highlights of Clinton Medicare Plan," 1999).
How much more will be cut in the future?

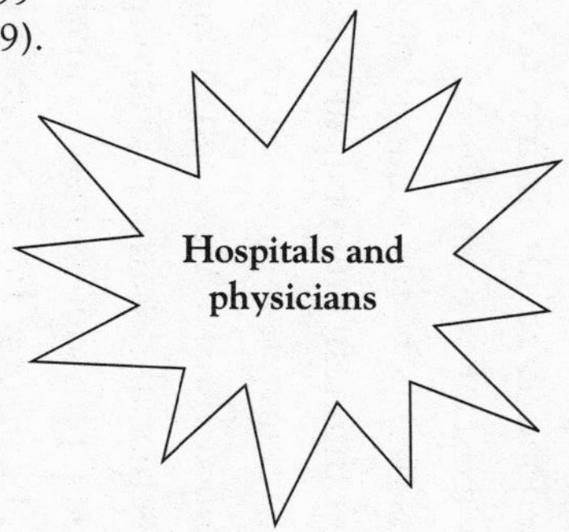

Managed care

Consumer demand and a booming economy have allowed a shift in enrollment from gatekeeper to open-access forms of managed care (Hudson, Haugh, and Serb, 1999).
Will this last?

Hospitals and physicians

Medical advances

Advances in gene therapy could radically alter how patients are treated.
How quickly will advances occur?

Niche players

Dr. Regina Herzlinger argues that "the guy who has a narrower range of mission is bound to be better than you are" (Meyer, 1998).
Will "focused factories" continue to grow and develop?

therapy technology, has to consider the likely timing of future introductions of effective gene therapies. Will an investment in cancer care have a useful life of three years? five years? The answer could change the willingness to invest on the part of the decision makers in a system. Without such investment, a system could not support state-of-the-art cancer care, and what would a system or hospital without oncology services be like?

The Impact of Uncertainty on Strategic Planning

Uncertainty confounds the planning process by invalidating the rules of the game under which the industry has operated, without revealing obvious new rules. This lack of direction (rules) increases discomfort and frequently results in a perception of greater risk than what actually exists. For example, many providers established managed care plans that not only required new management skills and operated under different rules but also assumed the responsibility for extending an uncertain amount of care for a certain price, thus increasing their real risk. Although management paid lip service to absorbing actuarial risk, the magnitude of the losses generated by many of these provider-sponsored managed care initiatives was unexpected. The assumed risks extended beyond the narrow focus of providers' investments. Many providers failed to realize that "the risks of getting into managed care include not only the potential of direct losses that must be replaced by cash reserves but possible contamination of the parent system's credit rating" (Moore, 1999b, p. 2).

Uncertainty further confounds the planning process by clouding strategic imperatives. Management and board members of many health care organizations developed strategies based on the perceived "certain" futures described in Table 1.1. As these assumptions failed to materialize, organizations often were left with strategies ill-suited to the resultant environments, but they refused to acknowledge their failure and develop alternative strategies. A good example of this is primary care practice acquisition. Many hospitals acquired primary care because of the assumption that gatekeeper models of managed care could and would channel patients to selected providers. Most of them have since experienced significant losses in their primary care practices and, with the decline of the gatekeeper model of care, have not enjoyed the benefits of channeling (Peters, 1999). In 2000, many organizations are continuing to allocate considerable resources in an attempt to make their physician practices profitable, without first addressing the question of whether it still makes sense to own practices at all.

Traditional Approaches Fail to Address Uncertainty

According to Michael E. Porter, "every firm deals with uncertainty in one way or another. Uncertainty is not often addressed very well in competitive strategy formulation, however" (1985, p. 18). Traditional strategic planning approaches often failed to adequately incorporate uncertainty because they approached it in a "binary" way of thinking, that is, seeing the world either as certain and predictable or as uncertain and entirely unpredictable (Courtney, Kirkland, and Viguerie, 1997). Neither approach develops strategies well suited for the dynamic, uncertain health care environment.

"The World Is Certain"

Organizations that think or want to believe in a world of certainty typically develop a single vision of the future and then craft appropriate, discrete strategies to succeed in the future envisioned. This approach to planning downplays the presence of uncertainty, often by averaging out uncertainties in order to develop a "most likely" future scenario. By doing so, they develop a vision and strategies that may not reflect the future environment in which they will operate. Organizations accustomed to approaching the future as one knowable outcome often find it difficult to create a new culture that is able to embrace, or even recognize, uncertainty.

"The World Is Uncertain"

At the other extreme, some organizations tend to think that right now everything is uncertain; therefore they question the value of planning. This attitude is especially prevalent in those organizations disappointed with or disillusioned by the results of their strategic initiatives over the past five years. The danger of this approach is that it frequently leads to one of two equally dysfunctional courses of action: (1) to abandon analysis and base strategies on instinct, or (2) to be so overwhelmed by uncertainty as to develop strategic paralysis.

Organizations that rushed to invest in primary care practices before such practices were bought by competitors exhibited behaviors consistent with the former response. Members of many system boards have been unpleasantly surprised to learn that their organizations invested in primary care practices not to expand market share (as they understood the intent); instead, the systems in effect purchased and now subsidize their own primary referral sources.

Organizations that have adopted wait-and-see plans are examples of the latter course of action (or in their case, inaction). Many organizations have focused recent efforts only on improving existing operations by reengineering. In doing so, they have successfully cut costs and streamlined processes but nonetheless seen their financial positions erode thanks to lack of a long-term vision or cohesive strategy for managed care positioning.

Ramifications on Planning

If uncertainty is a given and traditional approaches to strategic planning do not adequately address uncertainty, then new planning approaches, tools, and processes are required. This book focuses on updating traditional planning techniques, where appropriate, and introducing new techniques that address uncertainty more effectively so that health care organizations can develop dynamic strategies and cultures that meet the challenges of an uncertain health care environment.

A Framework for Conceptualizing Risk and Uncertainty

By understanding more about uncertainty and what causes it, managers can begin to combat the binary approach to thinking about uncertainty. There are varieties and varying degrees of uncertainty, and properly assessing its level assists health care organizations in quantifying the risks they take and developing strategies better suited to uncertain environments.

What Is Risk? What Is Uncertainty?

Although related, uncertainty and risk differ. *Uncertainty* is defined as the condition of being uncertain, or doubt; *risk* is the probability of loss. In true uncertainty, it is impossible to imagine all potential outcomes or assign probability to any one particular outcome. With risk, by definition, it is quite possible to assign a probability to a particular outcome.

Information, where available, can help one move from uncertainty to risk—that is, from being in doubt to knowing the odds. Organizations confronting profound uncertainty may reduce some of the perceived unknowns by obtaining and using credible **data.** However, as discussed later in this chapter, not all uncertainties can be eliminated by information.

What Are the Sources of Uncertainty?

To develop strategic planning approaches that accept and address uncertainty, it is important to understand its basic sources. As illustrated in Figure 1.2, uncertainty can arise from any of five sources: demand structure, supply structure, competitors, externalities, and time (adapted from Wernerfelt and Karnani, 1987).

Demand Structure

First, uncertainty can arise from not knowing what the future market will be, including the overall size of a market or how it will be segmented. For example, a hospital with an open-heart surgery

Figure 1.2. Sources of Uncertainty.

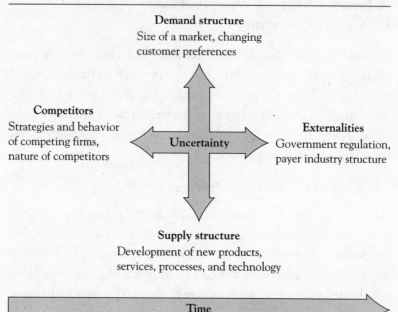

Demand structure
Size of a market, changing
customer preferences

Competitors
Strategies and behavior
of competing firms,
nature of competitors

Uncertainty

Externalities
Government regulation,
payer industry structure

Supply structure
Development of new products,
services, processes, and technology

Time

program that is considering upgrading or expanding its surgical and
intensive care capabilities needs to consider clinical advances in
less-invasive approaches such as intracoronary stents and radiation
and transmyocardial laser revascularization. If the less-invasive
approaches cannibalize coronary bypass surgery, open-heart surgery
volumes decrease significantly and demand for operating rooms and
intensive care beds can decline. The hospital faces uncertainty in
the ability to amortize its investment in open-heart surgery, even if
the total number of invasive cardiac procedures performed at the
hospital increases.

Supply Structure

Second, uncertainty can arise from changes in how products or
services are supplied or provided. Such structural changes can result
from unforeseen adaptations of internal operations as well as from

developments in technology. For example, many urban health care providers expected that there would be an adequate supply of trained, experienced individuals to staff operations. Many providers are now dealing with a shortage of qualified staff, not just in nursing but at all levels. To address these shortages, providers are enhancing on-site training programs and reevaluating traditional approaches to care delivery.

A parallel example from another industry may further illuminate health care's staffing supply dilemma. Consider how the role of and expectations for a cashier have changed. Twenty years ago, cashiers generally were expected to recognize a product, ring up the price marked on it, and give the customer the correct change, even if the process required subtracting. Today's cashier at a fast-food restaurant is no longer even expected to translate a verbal order into words on cash register buttons. He or she translates the order into a picture or icon that automatically rings up the correct price. Today no fast-food cashier needs to determine what change a customer is owed; the register computes it for the employee. Some chains have even eliminated the need for the cashier to count out the correct coinage. A fast-food chain requiring a cashier with yesterday's skill set could not compete in today's labor market. Those who gambled correctly on the systems that support today's employees gained competitive advantage.

Competitors

Third, uncertainty can arise from not knowing how your competitors will act, or from not being able to predict who your future competitors will be. For example, in Pittsburgh in 1999, Highmark Blue Cross Blue Shield proposed to finance the purchase by West Penn Health System of the failed AHERF hospitals. If yours is another system or hospital in the city, by traditional thinking is your hospital competitor now an insurer—one that says it will have no say in operations (Robinet, 1999)? Is the traditional insurer now de facto a competing provider?

Externalities

Fourth, uncertainty can arise from such externalities as government intervention and social norms or societal pressures. These uncertainties generally are the least controllable and can cause major changes to occur rapidly. For example, many states have certificate-of-need (CON) rules that regulate provision of selected services. Planning in a state such as Florida, which as of the end of 1999 had CON legislation in place, would be vastly different if CON requirements were eliminated. Overnight, profitable services that have been protected by the CON franchise could face price pressure, as they become subject to increased competition from new market entrants.

Time

Jeffrey Williams, who writes on business strategy, has said that "the significance of time in business goes beyond the reality that markets and companies are moving faster. There is a more interesting force at work. Business time is not only speeding up—business time is splitting markets apart, as well as the companies that compete within them" (1998, p. 1).

The final source of uncertainty originates in not knowing when and how fast a phenomenon will occur. Further, the parts of a health care organization face different strategic imperatives brought about by such issues as advances in technology and economic pressures. In 1998, the economics of home care were radically altered by changes in Medicare reimbursement. Systems with home health agencies faced a financial imperative to plan more quickly for home health services than for their other services.

The Level of Uncertainty

It is essential to differentiate levels of uncertainty based upon the extent to which it is possible to know of or understand an aspect of the future. Although there are no facts about the future, some aspects are clearer than others. A common framework classifies uncertainty into three levels: clear trends, unknowns that are knowable, and residual uncertainty (Courtney, Kirkland, and Viguerie, 1997). The extent to which an outcome can be understood ultimately determines its level of uncertainty.

Clear Trends

The future may be uncertain, but there are usually some **clear trends** that are knowable, easily researchable, and generally predictable. For example, population trends three to five years out can be predicted with a relatively high degree of accuracy. In addition, there are some less statistical trends that also are fairly safe to project. For example, assuming that there will be continued downward pressure on health care payment rates is a fairly safe assumption. We may not all agree on the exact form payments will take, but most of us would agree that prices are unlikely to increase in the near future.

Unknowns That Are Knowable

Unknowns that are knowable represent a level of uncertainty for which, if the right kinds of analysis are completed, the probability of certain outcomes can be assigned. In other words, the unknowns (uncertainties) become knowns (risks). Examples include consumer preferences, demand trends, and payer strategies. Companies in other industries spend considerable resources on market research and market intelligence to understand such unknowns and reduce business risk. Our experience is that many health care organizations are not willing to allocate resources for this kind of research. By default, they accept and assume greater levels of business risks than their counterparts in the corporate world do.

Leaders of health care organizations often say, "We know our customers (or markets, or competitors)." All too often, these statements are based on individual opinion or anecdotal evidence and do not adequately address the uncertainty inherent in the planning process. As outlined in Chapter Three, proper market research is essential to identifying, quantifying, and minimizing the risks an organization faces. As such, it also is important in developing strategy.

As an example, a large community hospital in a metropolitan market decided that it should affiliate, believing that its leaders knew the best affiliation partner on the basis of personal relationships and historical reputation. After conducting some primary market research on market position, organizational values and mission, clinical programs, and financial position, the hospital's management came to realize that they lacked an objective view of the strengths and weaknesses of each potential partner. The supposedly ideal partner identified by the organization prior to its market research had significant financial issues that excluded it from consideration as a viable affiliate.

Residual Uncertainty

The final level is termed **residual uncertainty.** Externalities and timing are prime sources of this level. Such uncertainties cannot be researched away, which leaves no basis on which to predict the future. Examples are the U.S. business cycle and its impact on health care, or the influence that consumer choice has on the future of health care.

Research related to residual uncertainty may not yield definitive answers. In some cases, organizations can pinpoint two or three alternative futures but cannot assign a probability to each. In other cases, a specific alternative cannot be predicted, but it is possible to bracket uncertainty and consider a range of possible outcomes.

Since residual uncertainties may cause discomfort, fear, or stress, the organization must assess an issue's strategic importance. Does a particular residual uncertainty pass the "so what" test? If so, then the organization should address this key uncertainty explicitly in its planning process.

Residual uncertainty often migrates to lesser levels of uncertainty over time. For example, at first, speculation about Medicare reform is unfocused. However, as potential reform proposals are presented and debated, especially during comment periods, hints of likely outcomes become clear. At this point, health care organizations can research alternative outcomes and approach the issue as an unknown that is knowable.

Conceptualizing Risk and Exposure

Because traditional planning techniques typically ignore uncertainty, they fail to give the organization adequate understanding of the degree of risk it is assuming and the sources of this risk.

Prudent Risk Taking

After assessing the levels of uncertainty it faces, an organization must decide on a course of action. This decision de facto means selecting a preferred level of risk. Dangerously, most people view risk as associated with change. It is important to recognize that an organization also faces risk from the actions it does *not* take, or from perpetuating the status quo. One hospital refused to discuss joint-venture development of a outpatient surgery center with its medical staff because the executives viewed the center as controversial and risky. Several surgeons made it clear that although they thought a venture with the hospital was best for everyone, they were going to pursue developing a center with or without the hospital. In this case, the far riskier course of action for the hospital was to seek to maintain the status quo, thus risking losing volume to the physicians' new ambulatory surgery center and creating ill will with the medical staff.

Exposure

Health care organizations tend to think of each risky action individually. Given the traditional approach to capital budgeting, a surgery center usually is considered a separate risk from an advertising campaign. In actuality, the risk the organization faces reflects its collective actions. This overall risk of the organization is called *exposure*.

The investment bank J. P. Morgan operates in constantly changing international financial markets marked by a high degree of uncertainty. To grapple with risk, J. P. Morgan produces what is called the "4:15 Report." Every day at 4:15 P.M., on a single sheet of paper, J. P. Morgan analysts project the company's exposure: the earnings worldwide that it has at risk of loss over the next twenty-four-hour period. Management then analyzes its positions, assesses the sources of risk, and, based on market prices, calculates a probability of loss.

Health care organizations cannot and probably need not calculate such a figure daily, but in an era of uncertainty a system or hospital must consider how much of its strategic budget and capital plan are at risk and to understand the implications of being wrong. Traditional planning approaches fail on both counts. Assessing risk exposure can be done properly only by linking strategic and financial planning; this linkage is discussed in Chapter Eight.

It is also helpful to identify and assess the major sources of risk the organization faces. For this, the scenario planning techniques discussed in Chapter Five are extremely valuable. For example, an organization may find that most of its strategies depend on the market moving in one linear direction. If so, this greatly increases the risk the organization faces. Even though the market may move in the expected direction, the movement often is not linear, causing strategic doubts or setbacks. By understanding the sources and levels of risk that it faces, a health care organization is better able to develop prudent strategies.

The Impact of Uncertainty and Risk

Developing better techniques that assess uncertainty, quantify risk, and lead to prudent strategies is only half of the story. Organizations and organizational cultures must also adapt in order to accept and respond to uncertainty. In their landmark examination of the firm, Cyert and March claim that organizations try to avoid uncertainty rather than confront it (Wernerfelt and Karnani, 1987). The best strategic planning can be undone by fearful, closed organizational cultures. Consider the following examples.

Example One: Auto Insurance Pricing

Insurance companies set premiums for automobile coverage according to a sophisticated actuarial analysis of several factors, one of which is geography. A car parked in New York City has a greater statistical risk of being stolen than the same car parked in Des Moines. Thus, the insurance company charges the New York City resident more for comparable insurance than it does the Des Moines resident.

To create an example, say a New Yorker who wants to pay lower insurance premiums claims to be a resident of Des Moines. The insurance company agent fails to check residency and sells the New Yorker the policy at a lower rate. As a result, the agent puts the insurer at economic risk despite the insurer's efforts to assess, quantify, and develop a strategy to adjust for different levels of risk. Further, if the insurer has inadequate monitoring processes in place, the risk is unrecognized until the policy holder files a claim for a stolen car.

Example Two: Clinical Protocols

A hospital and its largest cardiovascular medical group developed a clinical protocol that identified specific medical devices to be used. Both sides agreed that the protocol improved quality of care and cost efficiency. The hospital entered into contracts with payers on the basis of costs associated with this agreed-upon protocol. After a year, the hospital generated significant losses on the contracts in large part because of noncompliance with the protocol. It turned out that a second, smaller cardiovascular medical group, not directly involved in the protocol planning, did not support the selected protocol and continued to use the more expensive medical devices it favored.

In this example, the hospital's financial analyses and managed care strategy were appropriate, but the hospital put itself at financial risk because it did not develop a monitoring plan to ensure compliance.

Example Three: Service Line Planning

Sixteen surgeons approached a hospital asking for financial support for a freestanding surgery center, for which the physicians submitted a CON application. The hospital declined the request because it felt there was no need for a second center, given that the hospital had its own recently remodeled ambulatory surgery unit. In addition, the physicians did not want to give the hospital a say in operations, even though it was being asked to supply half of the financing. In working with the surgeons, the hospital realized that the physicians' real issue was frustration with inefficiencies in operation of the hospital's ambulatory surgery unit. By agreeing to overhaul areas such as scheduling and staffing, the hospital convinced eleven of the surgeons to pull out of the group supporting a new center.

Summary

These three examples illustrate that dealing with uncertainty involves much more than assessing uncertainty, assigning probability, and calculating financial risk. Successful organizations need to develop organizational cultures that are able to respond quickly, and willing to establish mechanisms that monitor implementation. These issues are dealt with fully in Chapter Nine.

Conclusion

It would not be enough for J. P. Morgan simply to recognize that uncertainty and risk exist. The company takes steps daily to respond to the risks it faces by developing and altering strategies over time to minimize or exploit risk. Similarly, understanding uncertainty and risk is just a first step for health care organizations. It is critical for success to develop planning processes and tools that address uncertainty in the planning cycle and to strive for an organizational culture responsive to risk. Chapter Two begins the work of developing effective strategic planning processes by identifying aspects of traditional planning approaches that are useful, those aspects requiring modification, and those that must be augmented with new tools.

Lessons Learned

✓ Uncertainty is a reality in health care.

✓ Traditional planning approaches inadequately address uncertainty. As such, organizations that rely on these techniques and processes face the danger of developing strategies that place them at too much risk, of not having appropriate monitoring devices to stay in step with future developments, and of fostering an organizational culture unable to recognize and capitalize on uncertainty.

✓ The future is neither certain nor wholly unknowable. There are shades and nuances of uncertainty and risk in all future events and potential outcomes.

✓ Uncertainty can be managed to some extent by understanding its core sources and carefully assessing what levels of uncertainty exist.

✓ The degree of risk that an organization assumes is influenced significantly by its approach to planning. Inadequate planning or improper implementation can put any organization at great strategic or financial risk.

2

Strategy Formulation in Health Care

Susanna E. Krentz and Janet S. Young

Will today's health care organizations be ready to compete in tomorrow's world? What new tools and techniques can be incorporated into the process to turn planning into strategy setting? This chapter gives an overview of strategy formulation in health care organizations, including a critique of traditional planning approaches. We also identify and discuss aspects of traditional strategic planning, both those that remain valuable and those that should be modified or enhanced given the uncertainty of the changing health care environment.

Health Care Planning

As do their counterparts in other industries, health care organizations engage in strategic planning processes to define future direction and to develop a framework for allocating resources and effort. Ideally, the strategic planning process promotes attaining **goals** that fulfill a company's **core purpose** and values, and results in an improved financial position. For industries such as health care that are characterized by highly dynamic and volatile environments, strategies that fulfill organizational purpose and vision often become "moving targets," contributing to the complexity of planning activities.

The fundamentals of strategic planning are applicable to any business or industry. However, the health care industry is characterized by four unique factors that influence its planning processes.

Industry Restructuring

Over the past decade, efforts to restrain skyrocketing health care costs have significantly contributed to a restructuring of the health care industry. Failed federal health care reform efforts in 1994 sparked a grassroots approach by the private sector to control rising costs. The vast majority of employers have abandoned traditional indemnity plans in search of lower-cost managed care alternatives. In turn, providers responded by creating hospital and physician networks and integrated delivery systems in an effort to leverage their collective interests in the contracting process with better organized payers. As Russ Coile summarizes it, "Beyond the current era of managed care, the concerns of consumers, a spate of governmental regulation, and new attitudes about health improvement are combining to fuel a fundamental rearrangement of the financing and delivery of health care in the United States in the twenty-first century" (Gilkey, 1999, p. 4).

Diverse Constituencies

Also influencing health care planning is the presence of diverse constituent groups, or **stakeholders.** The actions and reactions of payers, providers, consumers, private sector industry, and government all have contributed to the health care industry's current state of flux. The future will undoubtedly bring even greater uncertainty to this already chaotic industry. These various constituencies often hold contradictory views regarding health issues, contributing to the complexities of health care organizations' planning considerations. For example, physicians generally feel that clinical quality is what matters most, while payers are more interested in cost-effective care, and patients may focus on access and customer service. Getting all of these constituencies to agree upon any one course of action is clearly unrealistic, but savvy health care organizations know they must consider the wants and needs of each key constituency in developing their strategic priorities.

Oligopsony Market Situation

A third characteristic that contributes to the dynamics of the health care industry is the presence of an oligopsony (Greek "oligo" = few, "psony" = purchase of victuals) market situation, whereby a limited number of purchasers of care exert a disproportionate amount of influence on the market. Through their actions the largest collective purchasers of health care services, the federal government and a handful of managed care payers in each market, have demonstrated their ability to wield significant pressure. Health care providers in many markets have responded by discounting deeply, reorganizing service delivery, and experimenting with the assumption of insurance risk.

The Public's View of Health Care as a Right

Further influencing the planning priorities of today's health care organization is public opinion, which regards the rights of individuals to access to care. Despite the current insurance structure and nearly 44 million uninsured, the American public has generally held the view that unrestricted access to health care should be an inalienable right for all. Health care providers must remain sensitive to the views of the public regarding access to care issues, while understanding that the practical economics of unlimited access are not well understood.

The general uncertainty that looms over the future of the U.S. health care system is not surprising, considering the increasingly volatile market in which health care organizations of all types—systems and hospitals, managed care plans, physician groups, and niche players—operate. Financial pressures on health care organizations continue to intensify as payers ratchet down their payments. With reduced financial resources and capability, even greater uncertainty lies on the horizon, because organizations will have fewer funds with which to manage delivery of radically different modes of care in the twenty-first century.

Health Care Planning Through the Decades

The planning priorities and strategies of health care organizations have evolved over time to reflect the changing dynamics of the industry, as well as the broader-reaching economic and political climates of the United States. A review of historical planning priorities and strategies is helpful in framing the challenges presented by the uncertainty of health care delivery in the twenty-first century. In each era, planners in health care have adapted appropriately to the key constraints and market conditions they faced.

Post–World War II to Early 1970s

From the late 1940s through the early 1970s, the planning priorities of health care organizations were largely shaped by postwar economic expansion. The federal government increased access to modern hospital care with its decision to make construction funds for community hospitals available through the 1946 Hospital Survey and Construction Act, commonly referred to as the Hill-Burton program. Operating under capacity constraints and a "production" mentality, and aided by a government committed to realizing economic progress, providers focused their planning efforts on increasing physical capacity and improving availability of services to meet ever-increasing demand.

Facility planning was the focus of health care planners during this postwar era, and capital was readily available. From 1947 to 1971, the federal government disbursed $3.7 billion in Hill-Burton funds and generated approximately $9.1 billion more in local and state matching funds (Starr, 1982). The ensuing expansion of hospital capacity kept architects and facility planners in high demand.

Mid-1970s to Early 1980s

The 1970s were a time of rapid technological advancement in the field of medicine. At the same time that advances in technology were improving health care, they also were contributing to rising costs. Concerned with the escalating costs associated with new medical technology, payers pushed for increased regulatory control. The government responded with the National Health Planning and Resources Development Act of 1974, which resulted in formation of state health planning and development agencies (SHPDAs) and regional health systems agencies (HSAs), and introduction of certificate-of-need (CON) laws designed to establish and impose review criteria for planned capital investments.

Facility planning gave way to program planning during this era in health care, with hospitals rushing to develop services more quickly than their competitors. Because of the complexities of the new regulatory measures, many hospitals staffed their organizations with planners who were familiar with both regulatory compliance requirements and program planning techniques (MacCracken, 1998). Former regulators, not market-oriented strategists, set the standard for health care planning.

Mid-1980s to Early 1990s

Introduction of Medicare's DRG-based (diagnosis related groups) prospective payment system in 1983 created a new playing field for providers. Following the advent of this new payment mechanism, hospitals experienced an overall decline in inpatient utilization for the first time since World War II. With supply exceeding demand, providers adopted marketing orientations to help them preserve and build market share. Services were reorganized to create patient-friendly and cost-efficient environments. Planning in the mid- to late 1980s focused largely on business development strategies, with diversification of services becoming a key growth strategy of health care organizations. Corporate reorganization around diversification efforts consumed significant portions of senior management's time and attention.

As the 1990s approached, despite health care organizations' implementation of the aforementioned growth strategies and marketing tactics, they were faced with increasing competition and declining financial performance. Combined with the lack of financial success of previous planning approaches, financial vulnerability led the industry to focus on financially driven strategic planning (Jennings, 1998). In addition, the industry developed segmentation and niche strategies as part of an increased marketing orientation.

Mid- to Late 1990s

During the mid-1990s, market-driven reforms steadily supplanted failed government-mandated reform, making integrated delivery systems a key strategy of health care organizations. As managed care gained momentum, hospitals and physicians aligned forces, developing physician-hospital organizations to enable joint contracting for the anticipated capitation contracts with managed care plans. During this period, the number of independent hospitals dwindled, as mergers and acquisitions of health care organizations resulted in development of multifacility hospital systems. Physician practices were also subject to consolidation, with practice management companies and health systems moving quickly to gain control of these practices.

During this time, health care planners played a significant role in developing these integrated delivery systems and in other efforts to promote alignment of provider incentives among diverse provider entities.

The Future

Now, at the turn of the new century, the health care industry continues to evolve, presenting organizations with new challenges and opportunities associated with an increasingly uncertain and unpredictable environment. Emerging areas of focus include commitment to solidifying and enhancing the organization's core business, development of differentiation strategies, obsession with consumers, and strategies to address a market characterized by significant price pressures and intensified levels of competition. Effective organizations will successfully move beyond their traditional planning approaches, shifting their focus to strategy formulation that is integrated with resource allocation and financial planning.

Moving Beyond Traditional Planning Approaches

In general, planners in the health care industry have remained wedded to traditional textbook approaches to strategic planning processes; as Henry Mintzberg, Cleghorn Professor of Management Studies at McGill University, says, "Planning has always been about analysis—about breaking down a goal or set of intentions into steps, formalizing those steps so that they can be implemented almost automatically, and articulating the anticipated consequences or results of each step" (1994, p. 108).

Moving from Planning to Strategy

Thinking strategically differs in many ways from traditional planning. Figure 2.1 shows seven dimensions describing key differences between planning and strategy. Each dimension is not an either-or but can be considered a continuum. The two extremes of each continuum characterize the broad difference between planning and strategy formulation. For example, although the impact of successful traditional planning is generally incremental, successful strategy is more likely to result in organizational repositioning. Planning is more likely to be based on analyses and driven by consensus; strategy is framed by analytical concepts but accepts the notion that an answer often cannot be calculated or satisfy all needs and therefore requires leadership to drive the strategy.

Figure 2.1. Moving from Planning to Strategy.

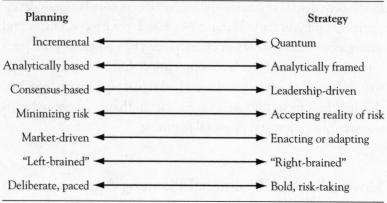

Planning	Strategy
Incremental	Quantum
Analytically based	Analytically framed
Consensus-based	Leadership-driven
Minimizing risk	Accepting reality of risk
Market-driven	Enacting or adapting
"Left-brained"	"Right-brained"
Deliberate, paced	Bold, risk-taking

Further, traditional planning seeks to minimize exposure to risk and therefore tends to respond to the market. Strategy is more willing to accept risk and take calculated risks, particularly if there is a desire to lead or enact the market. Traditional planning—with its analytical basis and consensus model—is comfortable for those who prefer a deliberate, rationally paced process. The conceptualization of strategy is often a better fit for those with an intuitive style, and it may feel bold and fast-paced (although still analytically framed). In both traditional planning and strategy under uncertainty, implementing strategies requires skilled management and analytical thinking.

Example: FedEx and the United States Postal Service

A comparison of two well-known entities, FedEx Corporation and the United States Postal Service, permits an organizational perspective to further illustrate differences between traditional planning and strategy.

FedEx, formerly Federal Express, typifies an organization that has embraced strategic thinking throughout its history. Beginning operations in April 1973, FedEx (http://www.fedex.com) pioneered the concept of a hub-and-spoke system for rapid small-parcel transport and delivery. The company's substantial investment in aircraft allowed it maximum control over flight schedules, creating an opportunity for the company to boast a level of reliability none of its competitors could match. FedEx was also able to achieve significant cost efficiencies over its competitors through its uniquely organized distribution system. Today, the company is thriving and remains ideally positioned to take advantage of global business trends in shipping and logistics.

In contrast, the United States Postal Service (USPS; http://www.usps.gov) is an organization rooted in deep tradition and a local community focus. The USPS first recognized mounting financial and competitive pressures following a decade of prosperity in the 1980s. In 1991, the volume of mail delivered by the USPS declined for the first time in fifteen years. The same year, recognizing that competition was steadily growing for each of its postal products, the USPS realized the need to reorganize its services. Seeking to preserve market share and become more competitive, in 1992 the USPS began to implement a series of strategies geared toward improving its efficiency and customer service.

It seems clear that FedEx's vision was achieved largely due to the visionary leadership of its chairman and chief executive officer, Frederick W. Smith, who enlisted the support of a loyal base of employees and then successfully led the company down a path fraught with uncertainty. The bold strategies of FedEx, which have allowed the company to dominate the overnight parcel delivery business for twenty-five years, are characteristic of a company that can capitalize on a changing environment. In contrast, the USPS initiated its reorganization in reaction to mounting competitive and financial pressures. The reactive, market-driven reorganization of the USPS, and its incremental approach to planning, were characteristic of a conventional approach.

Defined Assumptions

The traditional approach to health care planning is based on a clearly defined, static set of assumptions. Health care planners who used the traditional method were able to select a most likely future and then develop the organization's strategy around it. With this defined-assumption approach, an unknown was assumed to have a most likely and highly probably outcome. This view of unknowns often results in either underestimation or overestimation of uncertainty, both of which may have unfavorable results (Courtney, Kirkland, and Viguerie, 1999). An assumption that overestimates uncertainty often leads to the Chicken Little "sky is falling" sense of panic, which may result in rash actions—or lack of action entirely—because the challenge presented appears to be insurmountable by any initiatives the organization can devise. Likewise, a static assumption that underestimates uncertainty can lead to a sense of complacency, particularly in successful organizations. As an example, the successful entry of such niche organizations as ambulatory surgery centers and specialty hospitals generally met with few meaningful barriers to entry levied by the area's successful hospital providers.

Valuable Aspects of Traditional Techniques

The new approach to planning, which is presented in detail in the chapters that follow, builds upon, rather than abandoning, the tools and techniques employed by traditional health care planners. Here are some of the traditional planning tools and techniques that remain sound practices, even in a future of increasing uncertainty:

- Conducting thorough research and environmental analyses

- Identifying the organization's own distinctive competencies as well as areas of weakness

- Identifying environmental opportunities and threats

- Identifying key strategic indicators, for example, profitability, value, investment in the community, service, quality

- Engaging in processes that incorporate views of diverse key constituent groups

Modifying or Enhancing Traditional Techniques

In contrast, some planning processes lose their effectiveness in increasingly uncertain or volatile environments. Among these are processes that yield strategies based on a single set of clearly defined assumptions, that yield inflexible strategies, and that work from an expectation that full consensus must be achieved prior to action.

In traditional planning practices, agreement among all participants is typically achieved prior to action. Expecting consensus among planning participants may impede strategy formulation or result in stagnation of the process altogether. Consider as an analogy that a verdict in a criminal case requires that a jury reach unanimity in its decision. The greater the level of uncertainty among jurors, the stronger the likelihood that they will be unable to reach a verdict. Similarly, as the level of uncertainty in the health care environment increases, so does the likelihood that organizations find dissension among planning participants. If consensus among planning participants is the expectation, the organization increasingly finds itself with "hung juries," paralyzing the planning process.

In an increasingly uncertain environment, planning participants must set aside conventional attitudes and approaches to strategy formulation. In the new era, the traditional view that planning priorities and strategies should preserve established and historically proven ideas no longer applies. Today's environment calls for planners to look beyond traditional approaches, focusing instead on innovation and creativity. Mintzberg asserts that "strategic thinking, in contrast [to traditional planning], is about synthesis. It involves intuition and creativity. The outcome of strategic thinking is an integrated perspective of the enterprise . . ." (1994, p. 108).

Linear Versus Fluid Processes

Because of faster pace and lack of predictability, there is also a shift in the way traditional planning and strategy are developed. The typical process for most health care organizations is to work through a straightforward, logical set of steps to develop a formal plan. Generally, this planning process can be described as linear, that is, there are defined outcomes that occur in a sequence. One step is completed before the next step is undertaken (Figure 2.2).

In contrast, when formulating strategy under uncertainty, the steps in the process are likely to be intertwined. Although the organization ends up with outcomes that can be labeled "the plan," its thinking and deliberations are not linear, but more fluid in nature. Whereas hospital planners under a traditional approach would first agree on the organization's mission, then define the vision, and move on to strategies, those in a hospital developing strategy in today's uncertain environment are just as likely to debate strategy before finalizing the vision. Only after issues have been examined from many angles do vision, goals, and strategies emerge.

Transferable Skills

As health care organizations move away from traditional planning and toward strategy development, the fundamental attributes of their planning practices also are likely to change. Moving along the continuum from traditional planning to strategy does not necessitate abandoning all of the skills and expertise developed along the way. In our experience, many of the skills used in traditional planning techniques are transferable to planning in an era of increased uncertainty. Here are examples of transferable skills:

- Developing sound methods for assessing the market and the organization's current position

- Developing assumptions about the future

- Relying upon values, vision, goals, and strategies in formulating the organization's strategic plan

- Developing action and financial plans to guide the implementation process

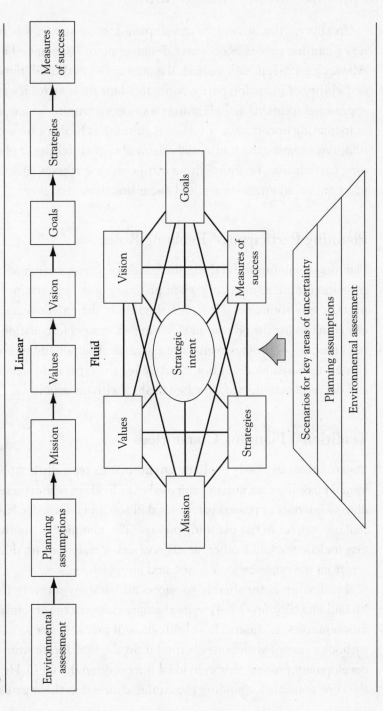

Figure 2.2. Linear Versus Fluid Planning Processes.

Linear

Environmental assessment → Planning assumptions → Mission → Values → Vision → Goals → Strategies → Measures of success

Fluid

Mission

Values

Vision

Goals

Strategies

Measures of success

Strategic intent

Scenarios for key areas of uncertainty

Planning assumptions

Environmental assessment

In short, "the answer to developing a good strategy is not new planning processes or better-designed plans" (Campbell and Alexander, 1997, p. 42); instead, the answer lies in the willingness and ability of planning participants to adapt their attitudes and approaches to traditional planning processes to prepare for a world of increasing uncertainty. To do so requires that health care organizations examine the traditional roles and responsibilities of planning participants, retaining those attributes that remain effective in an uncertain environment and discarding those that do not.

Planning Participants' Evolving Roles

Planning committees and the participation of a cross section of key constituents are as necessary when planning under uncertainty as in static environments. However, the role of the chief executive officer in driving the process and focusing on strategy formulation—not planning—becomes even more essential. Additionally, a broad consensus-based model is not effective for the types of leadership and decision making needed when dealing with uncertainty.

Traditional Planning Committees

Organizations in slowly evolving environments typically establish formal planning committees composed of individuals who represent diverse interests or possess particular skill sets and knowledge bases that are helpful in the planning process. The planning committee may include the CEO, other members of senior management, directors from the organization's board, and physician leaders.

Leadership is invaluable to successful strategy formulation. McGill and Slocum (1994) write that any new strategy an organization pursues, no matter how brilliant, will probably not succeed without someone with power behind it. In the health care strategy development process, this individual is most often the CEO. He or she is responsible for guiding the strategic direction the organization pursues and, inasmuch, is pivotal to the planning process. The CEO may assume titular leadership of the process, while shifting day-to-day responsibilities to another individual. Nevertheless, the CEO's participation and commitment to the planning process are essential. Above all, others involved in the planning process should view the CEO as a "champion" of the process, ensuring an adequate level of commitment from other participants.

Particularly in larger organizations, there may be individuals whose work responsibilities are specifically dedicated to planning activities. The titles of chief corporate development officer, vice president of planning, and director of planning are commonly used for individuals assuming leadership of the planning process in their organizations. These individuals usually report directly to the CEO and are responsible for guiding and managing the planning process. Other members of the organization management team, such as the chief operating officer, chief financial officer, and directors of business development and marketing, may also be included in the planning process.

Board members are often involved in the planning process as well. In most organizations, the board of directors is the formal authority whose approval is needed to endorse the fundamental strategic direction of the organization. Board members involved in the planning process often prove to be among the most valuable members of the committee thanks to their varied backgrounds; members may possess special expertise in another discipline, such as tax law, which can enhance the evaluation of contemplated strategies.

Finally, physician leaders round out the composition of traditional planning committees. The criteria used for physician representation on the planning committee depend heavily on the unique characteristics of the organization's medical staff—including its politics. For example, a hospital may seek to balance primary care and specialist representation on the committee, or it may choose to balance faculty and community-based physician representation.

Demonstrated leadership among the medical staff, such as involvement with hospital committees, is another commonly used selection criterion. Regardless of the criteria used, organizations usually attempt to make selections that represent the broadest cross section of physician interests possible, to build the medical staff's support of the planning process.

The number of individuals on a traditional planning committee and its specific composition vary according to a host of factors, including the organization's size, structure, and culture. Larger organizations may opt to organize larger planning committees to ensure ample representation of all key constituencies. If the organization is closely affiliated with or is a subsidiary of a larger organization, system representatives also may be included in the strategic planning process. In our experience, the best size for a formally organized planning committee that is expected to function as a true working group is twelve to fifteen members.

Planning Approaches and Committee Functions

Because of stylistic and cultural differences, organizations employ various techniques in their approaches to the planning process. Some prefer a top-down method, whereby strategies are developed at the highest levels and then disseminated through the organization. Conversely, some organizations opt for a bottom-up method of planning, in which strategies are developed at lower levels of the organization and pushed up for evaluation, decision, and implementation. Still other organizations use a physician-driven approach to planning, particularly if physicians have active participation in the organization's management or an ownership or other financial interest. In our experience, a bottom-up or grassroots approach is not likely to result in effective strategic decisions owing to the heightened complexity inherent in increasingly uncertain environments. However, these planning methods continue to be useful for routine program planning efforts.

In general, planning committees are responsible for evaluating, selecting, and recommending core strategies, as well as assessing proposed strategic capital expenditures. The specific functions of planning committees vary by organization, with availability of resources and varying degrees of interest among participants being key determinants of any single planning committee's distinct activities.

Although the composition, size, planning approach, and functions vary among organizations, four key traits are common among effective planning committees:

1. First, the committee enjoys visible top-management leadership and support.

2. Second, it exudes a proactive attitude that subsumes individual interests to those of the organization as a whole. This aids in building consensus among members of the committee.

3. Third, members share a clear understanding of their responsibilities and charge ("Strategic Planning Committees," 1997). Effective planning committees should be able to secure the support of board members and the medical staff.

4. Fourth, the committee members recognize that consensus does not mean unanimity; members must on occasion agree to disagree, and they also must be prepared to move on so as not to undermine the entire planning process.

Regarding this last point, there is a real danger in seeking unanimity of opinion. (This is discussed in greater detail in Chapter Nine.) A chain is no stronger than its weakest link; demanding unanimity often results in a lowest-common-denominator strategy prevailing, not the strategy that is best for the organization.

Changing Roles and Responsibilities

Though many aspects of traditional planning will be effective in the future, the individuals who are involved in the strategic planning process will be lost in a new era of increasing uncertainty if they are unwilling to modify their traditional views of planning. Individuals who are most comfortable and successful in planning under uncertainty will be responsive and willing to take risks; they will embrace the uncertainty of the future.

In the new planning environment, participants must possess several valuable traits. Topping the list are flexibility and creativity because, with increasing frequency, what has worked well in the past no longer translates into effective strategies for the future. Similarly, in rapidly changing environments, strong intuitive skills surpass the value of experience in relative importance. As illustrated in the case of the United States Postal Service, strategic stagnation occurs in organizations that cling to past ways of doing things and fail to place adequate emphasis on how things will be different in the future. McGill and Slocum adeptly summarize this point by arguing that using the "last war as tomorrow's guide"—that is, using past experience as a predictor of the future—is an inadequate organizational response in a rapidly changing environment (1994, p. 66).

Additionally, effective organizations seek out individuals with forward-thinking attitudes to take roles of leadership in strategy formulation. Health care organizations seek planning participants who are willing to take prudent risks and accept the possibility of failure. Individuals who are able to balance these key traits with well-honed analytical skills are highly marketable in an increasingly uncertain future.

Conclusion

As health care enters an era of new uncertainties, effective organizations are sorting through their traditional approaches to planning, preserving elements that endure and supplementing them with new concepts. To achieve effectiveness in this new era, organizations are finding that they must be innovative, since the value of experience as an indicator of the future diminishes as uncertainty increases. Also, organizations are realizing that there are no riskless strategies, and that leaders must acknowledge the level of risk they are undertaking and embrace change as they enter uncharted waters.

Finally, the leaders of effective twenty-first century health care organizations are taking responsibility for lighting the way toward a new planning era. They accomplish this by advocating for change from the status quo and by remaining a highly visible presence throughout the planning process.

To reiterate, many of the tools and techniques used in traditional planning processes, as well as the skills previously developed by health care planning participants, are transferable to the new environment. In fact, the best foundation for a new approach to planning is thorough understanding of today's strategic positioning. The next chapters explore in depth the new five-phase strategy cycle, which is illustrated in Figure 2.3. Readers who are familiar with the planning techniques currently used in health care organizations will observe that the first phase of the new strategy

Figure 2.3. The Five-Phase Strategy Cycle.

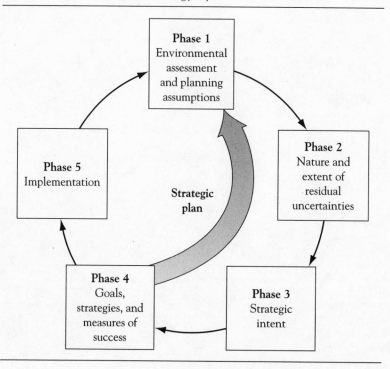

cycle contains planning elements commonly used in the planning processes of health care organizations today.

Lessons Learned

✓ In changing environments, past experience is no longer a good predictor of the future.

✓ Effective leaders advocate for change from the status quo and are highly visible during the planning process and implementation.

✓ Strategic planning must be led from the top.

✓ Consensus-based planning can result in lowest-common-denominator strategies. Rarely are such strategies effective.

✓ Many traditional planning tools and processes—namely, conducting thorough research, carrying out environmental analyses, and identifying key strategic indicators—are still valid and should continue to be used during strategic planning efforts.

✓ Effective organizations adapt to their changing environments by explicitly selecting the risks they are willing to undertake and by embracing change.

3

Reducing Planning Risks
Through an Environmental Assessment

Judith L. Horowitz, Tracey L. Camp, and Carrie S. Stahl

I s an **environmental assessment,** which focuses on the past and
present, relevant to planning in times of uncertainty? Do health
care executives recognize the importance of creating a culture in
which **strategic information** (not "data dumps") is expected, demanded, and used effectively? This chapter explains why a focused
environmental assessment is the foundation for effective strategic
planning and can help health care organizations adapt to the changing landscape of the industry. The iterative assessment process is
explained, demonstrating how to address an organization's unique
future challenges and opportunities. We also identify key components of the environmental assessment and give examples of using
graphics in conveying information.

Importance of the Environmental Assessment

An environmental assessment, also referred to in this chapter as a
situation audit, is a thorough review of the internal and external
conditions in which an organization operates. Done well, the environmental assessment serves as the backbone of the strategic planning process. It facilitates developing a common understanding of
the market, highlights the organization's historical and current position within that market, delineates clear trends for the future, and

identifies areas where uncertainty looms. Once completed, the environmental assessment serves as a platform for strategic decisions within the organization, as well as a benchmark against which progress can be measured. However, since senior leaders in health care frequently encounter data dumps masquerading as environmental assessments, many do not perceive the situation audit as adding authentic value to the planning process. As a result, senior management is often reluctant to invest resources in developing new assessments.

In today's health care market, the environmental assessment is an essential tool for reducing the risks associated with planning for the future. If expertly conducted, the situation audit assists leadership in identifying:

- What has worked well for the organization historically

- Its competitive position within the market

- The characteristics of organizations that will be successful in the future

- The key unknowns that will have an impact on the organization in the future and how these uncertainties can be addressed in the planning process

The assessment serves as the foundation for developing planning assumptions about the future. The great hockey player Wayne Gretzky understood the importance of anticipating the future and based the success of his career on it. He attributes his outstanding achievement not to his skating skill but to his ability to anticipate where the puck is headed on the ice and change his course accordingly. Like Gretzky, today's health care organizations need to be armed with information to help them "skate to where the puck is going." Of course, they also need to know where they currently stand.

The challenge, however, is that the past is becoming less and less reliable as a predictor of the future. The environmental assessment addresses this reality by introducing a mechanism into the planning process whereby an organization can distinguish between clear trends based on the past and areas of future uncertainty. The situation audit sets the stage for developing alternative strategic responses by uncovering the areas where uncertainty is greatest. For each area of uncertainty, a range of futures is possible, potentially requiring varied strategic responses.

As shown in Figure 3.1, the process of developing the environmental assessment and assumptions about the future is iterative. The first round of analysis affords a solid overview of both the market and the organization, resulting in identification of two principal sets of findings: clear trends and key uncertainties. From the clear trends, the organization can develop projections about the

Figure 3.1. The Iterative Assessment Process.

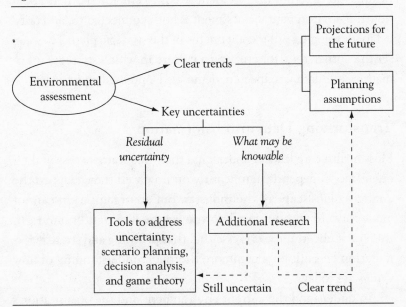

future without additional analyses. The key uncertainties must be further divided into two groups: those that can be clarified as a result of additional research; and residual uncertainties, which cannot be researched away. The residual uncertainties represent the greatest planning risks for the organization and therefore must be deliberately and carefully addressed by developing planning assumptions as part of the overall process. (Chapter Four includes specific examples of clear trends, unknowns that are knowable, and residual uncertainties. Chapter Five introduces various planning tools to address uncertainty, including scenario planning.)

The environmental assessment should be a required element of any strategic planning process. Health care executives must recognize that trying to develop a strategic plan without an environmental assessment is akin to trying to erect a building without a foundation. It is imperative that senior leaders recognize the value of the situation audit and play a visible role in building support for its importance as the foundation of the planning process. In many organizations, senior management needs to enlighten others about how the environmental assessment is both connected to, and critical in, developing other components of the strategic plan. They can set the cornerstone for creating a culture in which strategic information, not data, is expected, demanded, and used effectively.

Transforming Data into Information

Most health care leaders understand that the future success of their organization depends significantly on how well they adapt to the changing landscape of the industry. But an organization cannot move forward without first knowing where it currently stands. In this era of uncertainty, it is essential that planning and strategy formulation be built on a common, thorough understanding of how things are today.

To understand the current environment and the organization's position in it, many market and internal characteristics could be analyzed, potentially resulting in pages and pages of data. The challenge in the environmental assessment process is twofold: first, to identify what information is most important to support the decision-making process, and second, to effectively transform those reams of data into valuable information. Data are defined as facts that are organized for analysis or used to reason or make decisions. In contrast, information is knowledge derived from study, experience, or instruction.

Table 3.1 highlights the similarities and differences between data and information. Data and information both must be accurate and focus on what is most important to understanding the key strategic issues to be addressed by the organization. However, although data require translation or interpretation, information is structured to convey a message and support decision making.

Focusing the Assessment on Key Issues

A major objective of the environmental assessment is to identify and analyze key industry and market drivers that affect the formulation and likely success of alternative strategies. No organization can track every statistic or trend that may directly or indirectly influence its future. The availability of potentially endless data

Table 3.1. Differences Between Data and Information.

Data	Information
More is better	Less is more
Usually neutral	Can be positive, negative, or neutral
Generally not targeted to a specific audience	Should be tailored to a specific audience
Objective	Objective or subjective
Need interpretation	Conveys a message, leads to conclusions

necessitates making difficult decisions about the depth and rigor of the analyses to be conducted.

One efficient way to focus the assessment is to develop and test a set of planning hypotheses about major market forces. With these hypotheses in mind, a list of appropriate data elements can be compiled, and a set of analyses completed to test the hypotheses. For example, a planning team may develop the hypothesis that the providers in the market will consolidate over the next three to five years into three dominant systems. Accordingly, the environmental assessment could address such elements as current consolidation activity, provider market shares, financial capabilities of possible consolidators, and managed care penetration and contracting mechanisms.

Successful environmental assessments are intentionally limited in scope. In any industry, but especially within health care, there is no end to the material that can be assembled. But not all material, however interesting, is relevant to formulating the organization's strategy. The completed situation audit should relate a comprehensive story about the organization, unfolding a unified plot describing the past and present, while serving as the basis for developing assumptions about the future.

It is critical that organizations not fall into the trap of viewing the environmental assessment as an end in itself. Instead, senior leaders and planners should consider this activity as one essential part of a complex strategic planning process. The key to the success of the assessment process is deciding the appropriate level of detail to be examined. The goal is to build credibility in the information, while not overloading the planning participants. Additionally, constituencies within the process have differing information needs. For example, board members may prefer a high-level overview, whereas planning committee members may require in-depth formulation of the assessment findings.

Before completing any analyses, especially those likely to be complicated and time-consuming, the organization should ask,

"How will the outcome of this analysis affect our strategic decision making?" If the answer is "not much" or "not at all," the analysis is likely to be a waste of a valuable resource: staff time. The structure of the assessment should be driven by its primary goal, which is to present information to influence decision making and ultimately to affect strategy development. By presenting a compelling profile of the organization's environment, the assessment should heighten the planning participants' ability to construe relevant planning assumptions, envision alternative futures, identify strategic choices, and develop viable strategies for the organization to maximize its opportunities.

Potential Elements of the Environmental Assessment

The quality of the environmental assessment helps determine the utility of the ultimate product of the planning process: the strategic initiatives. To this end, it is critical to align the work of the assessment with the principal objectives of the planning process, that is, generating strategic questions, evaluating strategic options, and recommending specific strategic initiatives.

At the beginning of the process, it is important to select carefully those elements that are most appropriate in addressing the organization's future challenges and the resulting array of strategic opportunities. Accordingly, the data and information set for each organization are unique. However, most situation audits typically include four main components:

1. Qualitative information about the perceptions of the organization's key constituencies

2. Quantitative analysis of its internal environment

3. Data about the external market in which it operates

4. Comparisons to key industry benchmarks

Perceptions from Diverse Constituency Groups

To develop successful strategies in an era of uncertainty, an organization must evaluate itself and its marketplace from multiple perspectives. One way to achieve this is to solicit input from representatives of the major constituency groups that interface with the health care organization. Because senior management team members, department directors, physicians, current and former patients, payers, and the community-at-large all have direct relationships with the organization, they are a rich source of relevant and unique perspectives regarding the past, the present, and future opportunities and threats. These stakeholders can give valuable input to help the organization answer several types of strategic questions:

- What are their expectations for service?

- What elements of service do they value most?

- Why are some constituencies dissatisfied?

- What unmet needs can they identify?

- What do they think is necessary to succeed in the next decade?

- How do they perceive the image and reputation of the organization?

- How do they perceive the image and reputation of the competition?

Internal Assessment Elements

To understand completely an organization's position in the market, it is necessary to have comprehensive knowledge of its internal capabilities. The internal assessment is designed to identify the organization's specific strengths and weaknesses in key areas such as service mix, medical staff, and financial performance. Its ultimate goal is to impart understanding of the internal environment by highlighting aspects that influence strategy development. Table 3.2 contains a list of possible internal assessment elements, paired with the relevant strategic questions that each addresses.

External Assessment Elements

Assessing the organization's external environment results in understanding its relative competitive position, including opportunities and threats that may exist in the market. This analysis includes an overview of key market characteristics—such as demographics, market share trends, and potential regulatory changes—that may affect the organization's strategy. The external analysis also helps forecast future needs for health care services. Changes in technology, payer mix, managed care, and medical management can potentially affect how, where, and to whom health care services are rendered in the future. Table 3.3 contains a list of potential external assessment elements, paired with relevant strategic questions.

Benchmarking

Rising competition within health care is increasing the focus on continuously improving and outperforming the competition on as many dimensions as possible (quality, customer service, operating efficiency, and so on). As a result, health care providers are challenged to prove themselves as top performers meaningfully and measurably. **Benchmarking** can be a valuable tool in the assessment process, allowing the organization to compare its performance in key areas to that of competitors or peer groups. In a classical sense, benchmarking is used to identify best practices to gain insight and techniques for improvement in underperforming areas.

Benchmarks also are useful in developing detailed planning assumptions. Instead of basing assumptions on trends or forecasts, they can be developed based on performance gaps identified between the organization's own performance and that of the benchmark

Table 3.2. Internal Assessment Elements.

Element or Focus of Analysis	Key Strategic Questions
Inventory of Services	
Continuum of care	Are there gaps in the services we offer?
Core or distinctive competencies	Are there particular services that we should promote as distinctive competencies?
Facility and technological capabilities	Do we have the appropriate level of technology and type of facilities for the patients we hope to serve in the future?
Portfolio analysis	Should we "make" or "buy" those services in which we do not have a core competency?
	Should we reinvest or divest certain services?
Utilization Trends	
Inpatient and outpatient volume levels and average length of stay	How has our business shifted over time by patient care setting (inpatient, outpatient, home, physician's office), and is this the appropriate setting?
Service line strengths and vulnerabilities	In which service lines are we vulnerable to changes in use rates, physician practice patterns, managed care restrictions, and inroads by competitors?
	Are we capitalizing on those services where we are particularly strong?
Medical Staff Profile	
Specialty mix	Do we have appropriate specialty coverage for the population we serve?
Geographic distribution	Do we have enough primary care physicians to support affiliated specialists?
Activity levels, including physician dependency and loyalty	Do we have an adequate referral base and geographic coverage?
	Whom do we rely on most for our referrals and attending coverage?

Prevalent practice types	Are there opportunities to increase the loyalty of our physicians?
Age mix and dependency	Are we prepared to meet the practice needs of new physicians?
Board certification	Are we vulnerable in any particular specialty to physician retirement or downsizing?
	Is our medical staff adequately trained?

Financial Performance

Key financial ratios related to profitability, liquidity, capital structure	How well are we doing financially?
Financial capability	Do we have the financial capability to sustain operations and fulfill our mission?
Service line contribution margin and net income	Which service lines are most critical to our future financial success?
	For which service lines must we improve financial performance?
Case mix adjusted cost position	Should we reinvest or divest certain services?
	Is our cost position in line with our competitors?

Payer Mix

Dependency on specific payers	Upon which payers are we most dependent?
Level of managed care participation	Is our organization in appropriate managed care plans, given our patient population?
Dominant managed care payment methods	Are there opportunities to improve our relationships with payers and to share contracting risks and rewards?
Payer-specific contribution margin and net income	What is our payment level, and what portion is under our control? How should this affect our pricing strategy?

Table 3.2. Internal Assessment Elements, Cont'd.

Element or Focus of Analysis	Key Strategic Questions
Quality and Service	
Customer satisfaction and loyalty	In which clinical and service areas can we offer increased value to our patients?
Brand awareness	What is our brand awareness, and how can we improve or capitalize on it to address the organization's and patients' best interests?
Outcome measures	
Work Force Issues	
Vacancy and turnover rates	Have we successfully protected a valuable asset of the organization through adequate employee compensation, education, and professional development?
Average time to fill vacancies	
Compensation and benefit levels	Are there opportunities to improve productivity?
Employee satisfaction	
Productivity	
Skill level	
Professional development	

Table 3.3. External Assessment Elements.

Element or Focus of Analysis	Key Strategic Questions
Service Area Definition	
Based on patient origin, market share, and geographic continuity	From which geographic areas do we derive the majority of our patients?
	What populations are dependent on us for a large proportion of their care?
	Is the service area reasonably defined to include not only those markets where we have considerable presence but also those we would ultimately target serving?
Socioeconomic Profile	
Population projections (age, gender, ethnicity)	How will the population we serve today grow or decline over the next five years?
Household income and poverty levels	Do our service offerings match our population's needs?
Unemployment and educational levels	Are we adequately addressing the service needs of special populations (low income, elderly)?
Insurance coverage	
Community Health Status	
Mortality and disease incidence rates	How does health in our community compare to national *Healthy People 2000* goals?
Low-birth-weight and immunization levels	What potential interventions are needed in the local community?
Access to care	How can we improve the population's access to the health care system at the point of entry via our physicians and emergency room?
Availability of prevention and wellness services	Should we be in the business of prevention and wellness?

Table 3.3. External Assessment Elements, Cont'd.

Element or Focus of Analysis	Key Strategic Questions
Employer Profile	
Employer size and industry profile	Are there any health, wellness, fitness, or screening opportunities with local employers?
Insurance offerings	Should we be in the business of occupational health?
Size and scope of occupational health market	Should we pursue any opportunities to partner with self-funded employers?
Use Rate Trends	
Admission rates by service line and age	How much will the demand for inpatient services change over the next five years?
Trends in average length of stay	How do we expect our length of stay to change with increases in managed care and shifting of low-intensity patients to the outpatient setting?
Outpatient visit rates (ambulatory surgery, ER, observation, home health)	How much will the demand for outpatient services change over the next five years, and which type of provider will have the competitive advantage?
Market Share	
Trends by geography, payer, and service line	Has the organization's market position eroded or strengthened over time?
	In which areas are we the strongest, geographically and clinically?
	Are there opportunities for off-site service development?
Key competitors	Who are our key competitors by service and payer, and where have they made inroads?

Competitor Profiles

Key strengths and weaknesses and culture

How can we take advantage of competitors' weaknesses?

How do our financial performance and productivity compare to those of our competitors?

Geographic distribution strategies

Contracting and pricing strategy

Are our services priced competitively?

Utilization and market share trends

Are we vulnerable to encroachment by niche players for easily substitutable services?

Financial performance and productivity

Are we prepared to accommodate the boom in alternative medicine in our continuum by either entering the business or aligning with those providers already in the market?

Niche players and provider substitutes

How much has the market consolidated, and how will that affect our contracting opportunities and market position?

Integrated delivery system development and hospital consolidation or affiliation trends

Do market forces suggest a preferred approach to physician-hospital integration?

Managed Care Trends

Key plans and penetration levels by product

How large a player will managed care be in our market?

Should we pursue contracts with any new managed care organizations?

Prevalent payment methods

Are our contracts competitive with the market?

Financial indicators (medical loss ratio, premium levels, net income)

Is exclusive contracting likely?

Strategic focus (network size, open access versus gatekeeping, carve-outs and exclusivity)

Are we staffed appropriately to efficiently and productively manage under current and proposed contracting arrangements?

Quality focus

Are there care management initiatives we should implement to better align ourselves with managed care payment mechanisms?

Table 3.3. External Assessment Elements, Cont'd.

Element or Focus of Analysis	Key Strategic Questions
Physician Practice Trends	
Physician consolidation trends	Are we vulnerable to losing any key physicians to consolidation activity?
Ownership, affiliations, unionization	Do market forces suggest a preferred approach to physician integration?
Supply and demand	How does our physician complement compare to that of the market as a whole?
	Do our services and facilities match our physician partners' needs?
Legislative Environment	
Impact of Balanced Budget Act	What changes in regulations are possible?
Not-for-profit-status regulations	What would be the impact on us of any such changes?
Solvency, capital, financial requirements	What tax or other incentives are being developed that might affect strategy development?
Certificate of need (CON) and Medicaid changes	
Technological Environment	
New clinical developments	To what extent are existing technologies maturing?
Information system requirements	What are the significant trends and future possibilities?
	Are specific revenue streams vulnerable to new technologies under development?
	What alternative revenue streams should we consider as replacements?

organization(s). As with all tools, there are limitations as well as benefits to the technique. For example, benchmarking may foster a me-too mentality, rather than innovation. It targets the status quo, without addressing changing conditions and new market opportunities. Moreover, benchmarking typically focuses on operational issues, not the more critical strategic issues, and requires strict verification to ensure that measures are applicable and comparable.

Using Data to Reduce Uncertainty

In the previous section of this chapter, the list of potential data elements was discussed in the context of focusing the environmental assessment on information that is critical to decision making. In addition to identifying the types of data to collect and converting the data into useful information, another key to a successful situation audit is ensuring its effective collection and presentation. In this section we discuss the methodological issues surrounding data collection and reporting, including options for gathering qualitative and quantitative input and preferred ways to structure information to maximize its impact on the broad spectrum of planning participants. Additionally, this section highlights how information can be used as the baseline measure to monitor long-term performance against the strategic goals of an organization, by establishing an ongoing "dashboard of key indicators."

Qualitative Input: Market Research

Qualitative input is essential to a successful strategic planning initiative. Through qualitative market research, an organization can gain information on a spectrum of issues from its key stakeholders: senior leaders and managers, board members, physicians, payers, community leaders, consumers, and current or former patients. These constituent groups have a special interest in the organization and can give valuable input regarding its future direction and priorities.

In today's consumerism, health care organizations can learn much from other industries on how to monitor and assess opinions from increasingly sophisticated customer groups. By having a clearer understanding of the needs and wants of health care consumers, health care organizations can reduce the risks of planning for the future and increase the probability that strategic decisions are successful. Currently, many health care organizations conduct post-service patient satisfaction surveys. Very few initiate preservice assessments to determine consumers' expectations for service (although this is a very common practice in consumer product organizations). For example, when a car company plans to design a new minivan, it asks potential owners to describe the features most important to them and to identify their favorite colors and upholstery fabrics. Facing limited resources for expansion and new product and service development, health care organizations can benefit from this type of direct consumer input. Such feedback can be accomplished easily through focused market surveys that target a specific aspect of care or a specific product or facility. Facilitated focus group discussions and one-on-one interviews are other means to gather qualitative information about consumer preferences and the assumptions and feelings that underlie their opinions and perceptions.

A recent development in the realm of postservice surveys is a new generation of patient satisfaction surveys, such as those offered by the Picker Institute. These instruments target the dimensions of care that are of most concern to patients and their families (for example, access to care, coordination of care, physical comfort, and emotional support). In contrast, traditional surveys target the dimensions of care that are most interesting to the providers themselves, such as willingness of the patient to return to the facility and willingness to recommend the services to friends or relatives.

There are three principal ways to collect qualitative information: one-on-one interviews, focus groups, and surveys (either written or by telephone). Each approach targets slightly different audiences and works best in particular situations. However, in most cases, the choice of research method is based more on budgetary and time constraints than on specific methodological advantages or disadvantages. Table 3.4 highlights the benefits and limitations of the three methods for collecting qualitative information.

Typically, one-on-one interviews are conducted with management, board members, payers, and physicians, while focus groups are used with larger and relatively homogeneous constituency groups such as community leaders and former (or future) patients needing specific services. To focus on key uncertainties that should be addressed during the strategic planning process, during interviews we often use an exercise called Questions to the Clairvoyant (which is discussed further in Chapter Five). Although the exact form of the question varies, we typically ask interviewees, "If you could ask a clairvoyant—someone who can foresee the future—three questions about your organization, what would you ask?" How key stakeholders answer this question helps to identify the key uncertainties and risks that they believe the organization faces, and their responses can be used to focus data analyses and information sharing, as well as to stimulate group discussions.

Written and telephone surveys, which are an excellent way to gather a large amount of information from many people in a relatively short amount of time, are often used to solicit input from physicians and consumers.

All of these tools can be used to gather information on a variety of subjects, from perceptions of competitive impact and operational strengths to identification of opportunities for improvement and unmet consumer needs. Structuring the questionnaires and interview guides requires significant time to maximize opportunities for dialogue with constituents.

As an organization enters the environmental assessment phase, it should consider adding one or more of these qualitative research tools to its analysis toolkit. Valuable feedback regarding competition, relative strengths, and opportunities for improvement can be gained from these efforts. This information can then be used to

Table 3.4. Benefits and Limitations of Qualitative Input Methodologies.

Benefits	Limitations
Interviews	
More confidential than focus groups	Time-intensive; can be expensive
Generates greater depth of response, allows for follow-up clarification	Potential methodological inconsistencies if more than one interviewer
Can address issues of causality of perception	Interviewer can introduce bias to the process
	Responses represent relatively small number of participants because of time and cost constraints
	Respondents may not be honest if unsure about confidentiality of process
Focus Groups	
Group interactions tend to be more dynamic and spontaneous than one-on-one interviews	Limitations on the number of participants hinder generalization of results
Can address specific topics and issues meaningfully and comprehensively and explore rationale for responses	Requires skill and expertise for moderator to be effective
Results are verbal and qualitative, readily understood by leaders and planners	Typically, more expensive to conduct than surveys and interviews
Process can be accomplished relatively quickly	Potential for groupthink
Leaders and planners can observe groups in action to see nuances of expression beyond mere transcription of sessions	Not possible to explore topics in depth with each participant
Surveys (Written and Telephone)	
Can be customized to address needs and budget of those seeking information	Difficult to measure causality through survey methodology
Good way to get input from large numbers of internal or external constituencies	Process can be time-consuming
Efficient means to capture answers to a larger number of questions in a relatively short period of respondents' time	May result in response bias; only those most satisfied or least satisfied may be motivated to respond
	Low response rate may produce results not representative of targeted population

ground important strategic decisions in the realm of uncertainty. With such input, organizations can better plan for the future and deploy limited resources effectively.

Quantitative Input

Quantitative data elements also lend critical support to the planning process. The environmental assessment creates the means to combine vast quantities of data into a meaningful "story" that supports sound strategy development. In the age of the Internet, new data resources spanning the continuum of care become available daily. A mandatory early step in the environmental assessment is to inventory data sources already in place at the organization, so that gaps can be identified and filled.

With an ever-expanding number of potential data sources, however, it is more important than ever to assess the integrity of each and document its limitations. By acknowledging the underlying assumptions, limits, and biases of each data source, it is possible not only to identify the most appropriate and reliable sources but also to pose appropriate caveats in using the data. Some comprehensive sources of data can be costly, but many additional sources can be procured at reasonable cost from state and local agencies, regulatory divisions, and health care associations. Table 3.5 lists common examples of quantitative data sources, the types of information these sources can provide, and caveats for using this information.

Structuring Information

Once all the information for the internal and external assessments is compiled, the next challenge is communicating the information meaningfully to those involved in the planning process. Written reports including graphic elements become the workhorses for sharing the details of the environmental assessment. For the information to be useful, both words and exhibits must be easy to comprehend. When well-designed, graphics offer tremendous potential to focus participants' attention on key issues and options and to facilitate discussion and decision making. Graphics are unique in

Table 3.5. Quantitative Data Sources.

Data Sources	Type of Information	Caveats
State statistics (hospital association, state department of health, insurance commissioner)	Use rate, hospital market share, and charge data by product line, facility, age of patient, and payer gathered from patient billing records; utilization and financial data by managed care plan	Complete and accurate outpatient data are generally not available May not produce adequate use rates if the state does not mandate reporting or does not verify or audit information
Federal government statistics (National Center for Health Statistics, HCIA, Census Bureau)	Socioeconomic, utilization, and financial data across the health care continuum	Considerable time delay for reporting (2–3 years old) Data may be limited to Medicare patients
National information vendors (HCIA-SACHS*, Claritas, Inforum, Milliman and Robertson, SMG, CHIPS, InterStudy)	Utilization, demographic, financial, and managed care data across the health care continuum, from a variety of sources including proprietary claims databases, utilization models, consumer research, state and federal public databases, hospital and payer surveys, and professional associations	Can be very expensive Some components are based on black-box methodologies Some information is limited in detail
Professional associations (American Medical Association, Medical Group Management Association, etc.)	Operational, financial, and management statistics for physicians, nurses, and allied health professionals	Can be very expensive Some information is proprietary or available only to members Generally reliant on survey information, which can affect reliability and integrity
Websites (e.g., AHD.com [American Hospital Directory], InteliHealth.com, WebMD.com)	Health information, provider profiles, research studies, Medicare statistics, utilization comparisons	Some information may lack integrity or credibility Data available are generally less detailed

Note: HCIA and SACHS recently merged.

that they use images to portray quantities and relationships with clarity, precision, and efficiency.

Principles of Graphical Excellence

Graphics to represent relationships were invented about 250 years ago, after the development of logarithms, calculus, and the basics of probability theory. But in recent years, with frequent advances in personal computing, options for visual display of quantitative information have expanded dramatically. At present, it is estimated that between one and two trillion statistical graphics are printed each year (Tufte, 1983). But information design specialists complain that many computer-generated graphics fail to draw the viewers' attention to the sense and substance of the data, instead distracting the audience with the remarkable (but overwhelming) capabilities of the computer program itself.

Specific standards support clarity and excellence in displaying data. In *The Visual Display of Quantitative Information*, Edward R. Tufte states that "graphical excellence is that which gives to the viewer the greatest number of ideas in the shortest time with the least ink in the smallest space" (1983, p. 50). In essence, graphical excellence is achieved through well-designed presentation of interesting data and information, combining the distinct components of substance, statistics, and design. When graphical displays meet this standard, they:

- Convert data or perceptions into strategically relevant implications (see Figures 3.2 and 3.3 and Table 3.6)

- Communicate analyses requiring multiple assumptions in a logical fashion (see Figures 3.4 and 3.5)

- Portray multivariate information effectively (see Figures 3.6 and 3.7)

- Encourage the eye to compare and contrast different pieces of data (see Figures 3.8 and 3.9)

- Have a narrative quality and tell a story about the data using a combination of words, numbers, and pictures (see Figure 3.10)

- Display a large amount of data concisely and coherently (see Figure 3.11 and Table 3.7)

- Orient information spatially, as on a continuum or within the context of its geography (see Figure 3.12 and Table 3.8)

Dashboard of Key Indicators

The so-called **dashboard of key indicators** is a relatively new concept, wherein organizations can supplement traditional financial measures with criteria that examine performance on nonfinancial dimensions critical to their success (Kaplan and Norton, 1996b). An organizational dashboard of key indicators can be derived easily from the baselines identified during the environmental assessment, after goals and strategic initiatives have been identified. To be most useful, a dashboard process requires identifying an organization's strategic goals and objectives and then some collaborative decision making regarding the key indicators to measure performance toward the goals.

Even though it offers critical information along multiple dimensions, the dashboard minimizes information overload by limiting the number of measures used. There is no ideal number of indicators, with some organizations measuring as few as four and others as many as thirty to link their long-term objectives to short-term actions. Like the environmental assessment process itself, the unique circumstances of the planning organization suggest the most appropriate elements for inclusion as target measures of performance. For example, dashboard elements might include patient and employee satisfaction scores, market share growth, growth in the number of cases at a new ambulatory surgery center, number of covered lives in a managed care plan, length of stay in the critical care

Figure 3.2. Payer Mix.

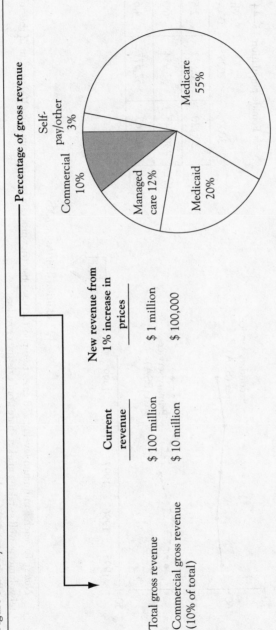

Percentage of gross revenue

Medicare 55%

Medicaid 20%

Managed care 12%

Commercial 10%

Self-pay/other 3%

	Current revenue	New revenue from 1% increase in prices
Total gross revenue	$ 100 million	$ 1 million
Commercial gross revenue (10% of total)	$ 10 million	$ 100,000

Note: By increasing prices just 1 percent, "Caring Hospital" can add $100,000 to its bottom line from commercial payers who pay based on a percentage of charges.

Figure 3.3. Fertility Rates.

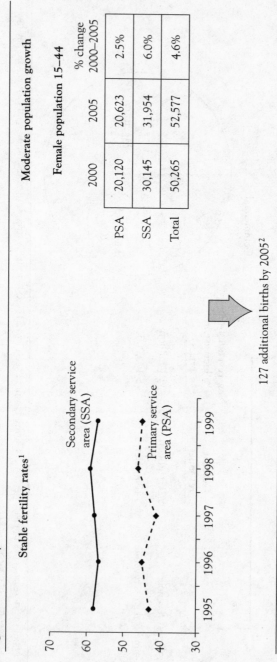

Stable fertility rates[1]

Secondary service area (SSA)

Primary service area (PSA)

70
60
50
40
30

1995 1996 1997 1998 1999

Moderate population growth

Female population 15–44

	2000	2005	% change 2000–2005
PSA	20,120	20,623	2.5%
SSA	30,145	31,954	6.0%
Total	50,265	52,577	4.6%

127 additional births by 2005[2]

Notes: To reach a minimum level of 250 cases to support a new obstetrics program requires capturing 100 percent of this incremental volume, as well as taking market share from existing providers.
[1] Births per 1,000 females aged 15 to 44.
[2] Assuming a constant fertility rate equal to historical five-year average (44 in PSA and 58 in SSA).

Table 3.6. Managed Care Customer Report Card.

Criteria:	How do health plans currently rate us? Current Grade	How would we like them to rate us? Targeted Grade
Cost	D	B
Member satisfaction	B+	A
Access to primary care physicians:		
• Hours of operation	B+	A–
• Practice open to new patients	B	A
Quality of care	B+	A
Flexibility in contracting	C	B
Data availability	C	B
Relationship with physicians	C	B
ER utilization management	B	A
Overall satisfaction	C+	A–

Note: To improve overall satisfaction of health plans with Caring Hospital, the greatest emphasis should be on reducing costs.

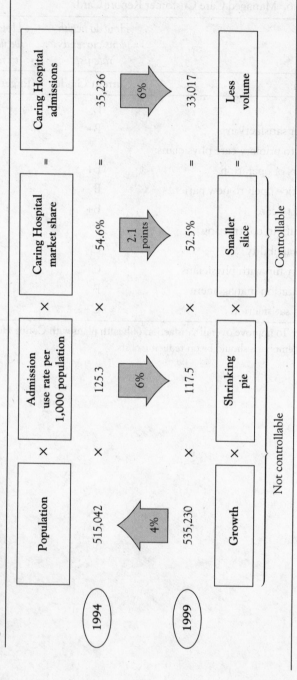

Figure 3.4. Fundamentals of Volume.

Figure 3.5. Physician Demand.

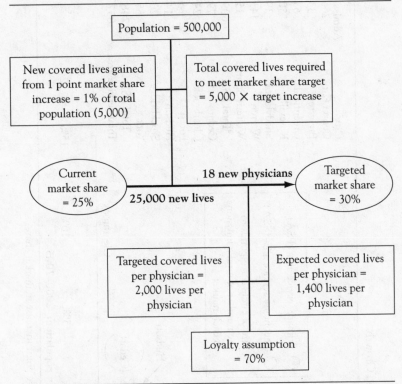

Note: To achieve the targeted five-point increase in market share requires adding eighteen new physicians.

Figure 3.6. 1999 Inpatient Market Share, Size, and Growth.

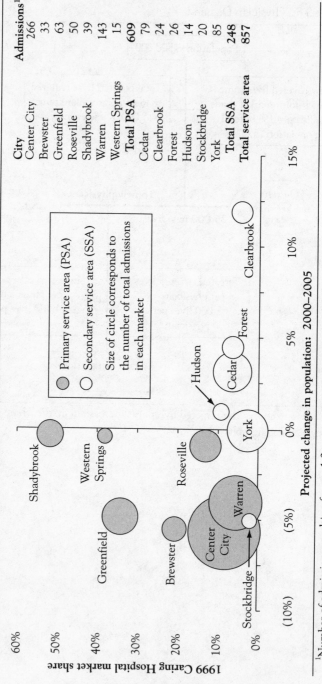

City	Admissions[1]
Center City	266
Brewster	33
Greenfield	63
Roseville	50
Shadybrook	39
Warren	143
Western Springs	15
Total PSA	**609**
Cedar	79
Clearbrook	24
Forest	26
Hudson	14
Stockbridge	20
York	85
Total SSA	**248**
Total service area	**857**

- Primary service area (PSA)
- Secondary service area (SSA)

Size of circle corresponds to the number of total admissions in each market

1999 Caring Hospital market share

Projected change in population: 2000–2005

[1]Number of admissions resulting from a 1.0 percentage point increase in market share

Figure 3.7. Socioeconomic Profile.

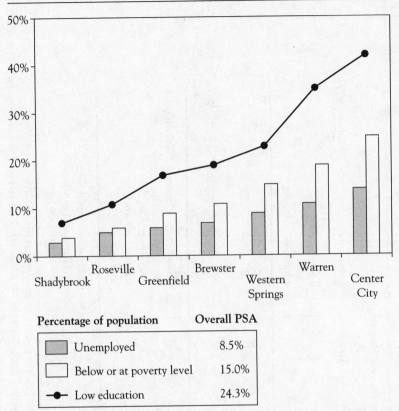

Percentage of population	Overall PSA
Unemployed	8.5%
Below or at poverty level	15.0%
Low education	24.3%

Notes: Low education levels are more closely linked with poverty than unemployment rates.

The unemployment rate is defined as the percentage of the population under age sixty-five who are unemployed. The low education rate is defined as the percentage of the population age twenty-five or older with less than a high school education.

Figure 3.8. Financial Profile.

Indicator	Caring Hospital Performance				Industry Median 1997[1]
	FY 1998	FY 1999	Trend	Comments	
Operating Margin	6.3%	3.2%	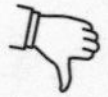	• Effects of BBA	N/A
Total Margin	8.9%	5.4%	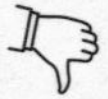	• Increased discounts	6.1%
Long-term liabilities to capitalization	34%	28%	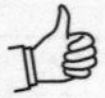		32%
Debt service coverage ratio	5.4:1	6.8:1	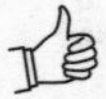		4.7x1
Days of net receivables	120	109	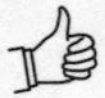	• If *days of net receivables* were reduced to the industry median, *days cash on hand* would increase to 79	63
Days cash on hand	60	30	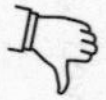		153
Average age of plant (years)	9.7	10.4	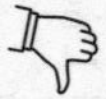	• $84 million would have to be invested to achieve the industry median	8.3

Note: [1] 1997 industry median is for urban U.S. hospitals with gross revenue greater than $150 million.

Source: Industry median data adapted from Cleverley, W. O. *The 1998–99 Almanac of Hospital Financial and Operating Indicators.* Columbus, Ohio: Center for Healthcare Industry Performance Studies, 1998, pp. 18, 60, 74, 84, 104, 140.

Figure 3.9. Admissions and Observation Visits.

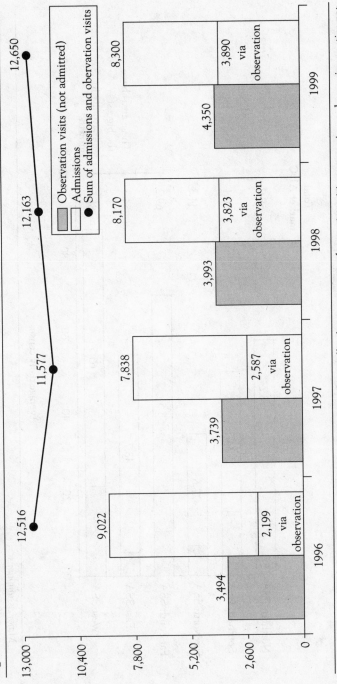

Note: Caring Hospital's declining admission levels have been offset by increases in observation visits, suggesting a change in practice patterns.

Figure 3.10. Projected Demand for Inpatient Services in 2005.

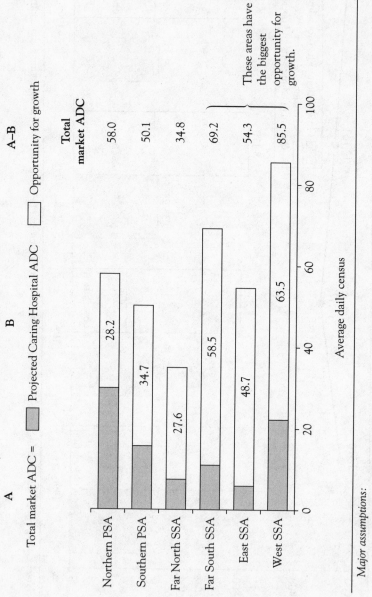

A

Total market ADC =

B   A–B

Projected Caring Hospital ADC   Opportunity for growth

	Total market ADC
Northern PSA	58.0
Southern PSA	50.1
Far North SSA	34.8
Far South SSA	69.2
East SSA	54.3
West SSA	85.5

These areas have the biggest opportunity for growth.

Average daily census

Major assumptions:

Admissions use rate projected to decline 2 percent per year
Population projected to decline in all areas
Length of stay projected to be 3.5 days in total market, 3.6 days at Caring Hospital
Caring Hospital market share projected to remain constant

Figure 3.11. Medical Staff Age Profile.

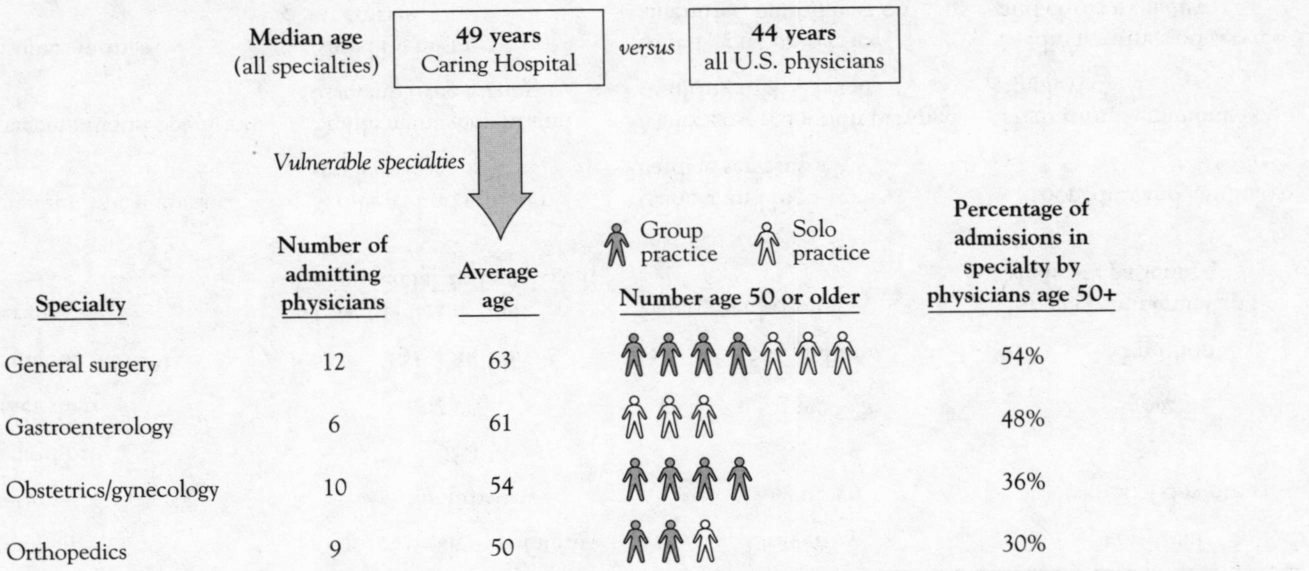

Median age (all specialties)		
49 years Caring Hospital	*versus*	**44 years** all U.S. physicians

Vulnerable specialties

Group practice / Solo practice

Specialty	Number of admitting physicians	Average age	Number age 50 or older	Percentage of admissions in specialty by physicians age 50+
General surgery	12	63		54%
Gastroenterology	6	61		48%
Obstetrics/gynecology	10	54		36%
Orthopedics	9	50		30%

Note: Caring Hospital has a relatively older medical staff and is vulnerable to potential physician retirement in several specialties (particularly those with many physicians in solo practice).

Table 3.7. Competitor Profile.

	Community Hospital	University Hospital	Big Bucks Hospital
Ownership	Not-for-profit, community	University	For-profit
Location	Suburban	Downtown	Outskirts of downtown
Licensed beds	380	825	323
Market share	25%	25%	20%
Net income (1999)	+$1.2 million	−$10 million	+$5 million
Payer mix	Low Medicaid; high commercial and managed care	Safety-net hospital	Targets commercial and Medicare patients
Strongest clinical areas	Women's and children's services	Cancer and high-tech cardiac services	Orthopedics and cardiology
Management and operations	Stable management and low employee turnover	Major cost reduction planned resulting in 400 layoffs	High turnover among employees
Consumer ratings	Rated highest on service amenities	Rated worst on service amenities, but highest on clinical quality of care	Medium ratings on service and clinical quality

Figure 3.12. Service Area Market Profiles.

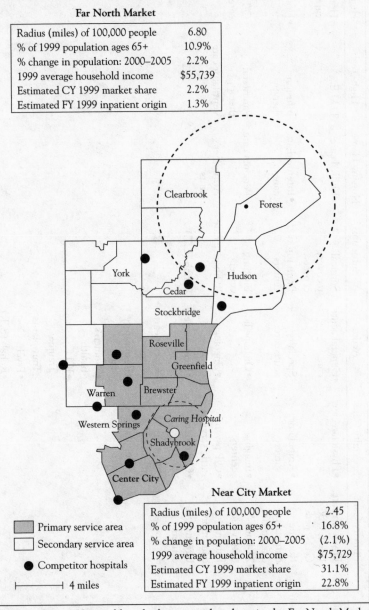

Far North Market

Radius (miles) of 100,000 people	6.80
% of 1999 population ages 65+	10.9%
% change in population: 2000–2005	2.2%
1999 average household income	$55,739
Estimated CY 1999 market share	2.2%
Estimated FY 1999 inpatient origin	1.3%

Near City Market

Radius (miles) of 100,000 people	2.45
% of 1999 population ages 65+	16.8%
% change in population: 2000–2005	(2.1%)
1999 average household income	$75,729
Estimated CY 1999 market share	31.1%
Estimated FY 1999 inpatient origin	22.8%

■ Primary service area
□ Secondary service area
● Competitor hospitals
⊢——⊣ 4 miles

Note: Caring Hospital has the lowest market share in the Far North Market, where the population growth is concentrated and where the age distribution is relatively young.

Table 3.8. Continuum of Care.

	Ambulatory Care		Inpatient Care			Home Care	
	Primary Care	Specialty Care	Acute	Subacute	Nursing Home	High-Tech	"High-Touch"
•Public health education	•Physician care (med, OB/GYN, peds)	•Physician care	•General acute care	Surgical recovery centers	Skilled care	D.M.E.	•Home health care (skilled)
Immunization	•Routine outpatient diagnostics	•Ambulatory surgery	Specialty acute care:	Brain injury centers	•Intermediate care	Infusion therapy	•Home aides
Research	•23-hour observation	•Imaging centers	•Orthopedics	Birthing centers	Personal care	Parenteral therapy	
•"Wellness" programs	•Patient education	•O/P psychiatric services	•Oncology	IP hospice care	Alzheimer's units	Ventilator care	O/P hospice care
Advocacy	Urgent care centers	•O/P rehab centers	•Neurosurgery	Rehab (L.T.)			
Industrial health		Sports medicine	Open heart surgery				
		Adult day care	•Respiratory care				
			•Women's health				
			•ICU				
			Trauma				
			Transplants				
			•Psych				
			•Rehab (S.T.)				
			•Substance abuse				

Note: • = offered by Caring Hospital

unit, and key health status indicators related to community benefit programs.

More and more organizations are implementing the dashboard process. The concept's principal appeal is that it fills a serious void in traditional management systems and constitutes a mechanism to monitor the progress of an organization's long-term strategy by measuring specific short-term financial and operational results. Additionally, the dashboard focuses managers on a handful of measures most critical to the organization's future success. The dashboard deftly focuses the attention of senior leaders upon global information rather than the details of the financial reports, thus greatly enhancing the scope and review of the traditional strategic planning process. For a complete discussion of developing measures of success, see Chapter Seven.

Conclusions

Market volatility in recent years has yielded a number of high-profile strategic failures. Current prognosticators forecast continued and growing uncertainty for the health care industry. Such uncertainty makes the environmental assessment even more critical as a means of reducing risk in the strategic planning process.

Many organizations are devoting insufficient effort to this critical component of strategy development. Unwillingness to devote resources to thorough assessment of the environment may reflect poor quality of past efforts, which often were compilations of unstructured statistics irrelevant to strategy formulation. Moreover, as the past has become less and less valuable as a predictor of the future, some leaders have concluded that the traditional assessment process is of limited benefit in strategy formulation.

It is precisely the information gleaned from the environmental assessment that is the key to moving an organization from the realm of uncertainty into strategic risk assessment. The discipline of the iterative assessment process allows industry trends to be differentiated from true uncertainties. The environmental assessment process is critical to establishing the organization's assumptions about the future in which it will operate. How an organization begins to envision its future through developing planning assumptions is the topic of the next chapter.

Lessons Learned

✓ Focused environmental assessments help reduce the risk of planning for the future by distinguishing between clear trends and key uncertainties. They are, therefore, a critical step in strategy formulation in this era of uncertainty.

✓ Environmental assessments identify and analyze key industry and market drivers that influence the formulation and likely success of strategies.

✓ Senior leadership must play a visible role in building support for and appreciation of the environmental assessment. They are also responsible for creating a culture in which information, not data, is demanded by management and board members alike and used effectively.

✓ Assessments should focus on relevant data and information that supports strategy formulation. Just because a data finding is interesting does not make it relevant to strategic decision making.

✓ Each assessment is unique, designed to address the planning organization's unique future challenges and opportunities.

✓ Health care organizations underuse accepted research tools to tap knowledge of the attitudes and expectations of increasingly sophisticated consumers. Consumer research tools are another means to reduce risks associated with planning for an uncertain future.

✓ A successful assessment is built upon a base of qualitative and quantitative input. Recent technologies have disseminated an array of new sources to satisfy every data need. Organizations must explore these options fully to find the most appropriate source.

✓ When transformed into well-structured information, data support the strategic decision-making and planning process.

4

Envisioning the Future Through Planning Assumptions

Cathy Sullivan Clark and Ryan S. Gish

W hat are planning assumptions, and why are they important? How does the reality of uncertainty affect their development? In this chapter, we explore these two questions about planning assumptions, highlighting the critical importance of planning assumptions during and following a formal strategic planning process.

What Are Planning Assumptions?

Planning assumptions are informed guesses about the future, serving as the critical link between the environmental assessment and identification of **strategic intent** and strategies. Because there are no facts about the future, all planning assumptions are by definition uncertain. Good planning assumptions, however, are not created in a vacuum but rather based on information from the environmental assessment. In developing planning assumptions, an organization anticipates its future environment and contemplates potential challenges, opportunities, and critical success factors.

Examples of planning assumptions are abundant. They range from the mundane (the sun will rise tomorrow) to the complex (the current rate of oil consumption will exhaust all reserves by 2050, dictating the need for an alternative energy source).

Even if he did not land in India, Christopher Columbus's discovery of the New World is a wonderful example of a planning assumption that was eventually proven correct. During the fifteenth century, European explorers traveled sea routes around the cape of Africa in search of silks and spices from the Far East. Assuming that the world was flat, they chose this route rather than proceeding across the Atlantic Ocean and risking death by falling off the edge of the world. In search of a new trade route, Columbus bucked conventional wisdom and sailed west from Europe, reaching what he believed to be the eastern edge of India. Implicit in Columbus's actions was his belief that the world was spherical rather than flat— a radical assumption for any fifteenth-century sailor.

The Walt Disney Company's experience in creating Euro Disney illustrates the danger of even the most sophisticated organization making flawed planning assumptions (McGrath and MacMillan, 1995). In planning for Euro Disney's opening in 1992, Disney made the erroneous assumption that Euro Disney "visitors," or guests, would behave like their American counterparts. Based on this un-informed assumption, they designed Euro Disney largely as a replica of Disney's American theme parks—and then experienced early financial losses from the new business venture. A comparison of Disney's flawed planning assumptions and the actual behaviors of guests is presented in Table 4.1.

Planning assumptions have been used in traditional health care planning for many years. Chapter One offered examples from the past of flawed assumptions about the future of health care, including the assumption by the American Hospital Association that hospitals and health systems would want to contract directly with HCFA through provider-sponsored organizations (PSOs). These assumptions, along with many others, missed the mark. Past failures, though, are not cause to abandon the practice of developing planning assumptions. What is needed instead is a new approach to developing planning assumptions, one that recognizes and actively incorporates the reality of uncertainty about the future.

Perhaps the biggest mistake in past development of planning assumptions was the tendency either to treat all assumptions as

Table 4.1. Euro Disney's Flawed Planning Assumptions.

Category	Planning Assumption	European Behavior	Why Was It Flawed?
Admission price	Guests will be willing to pay a premium to enter Euro Disney because it is *Disney*.	Guests balked at the $40 admission price.	When the park opened, Europe was in the midst of a major recession, causing many families to reduce entertainment spending.
Hotel accommodations	Guests will stay an average of four days.	The average stay was only two days.	Euro Disney had fifteen attractions, compared to Disney World's forty-five. Guests were able to visit all attractions in one or two days.
Food	Guests will "graze" all day at the park's many concessions.	Europeans flooded the dining areas at noon.	Europeans follow a much more programmed meal schedule than Americans. Euro Disney's restaurants, designed for continuous streams of patrons, were insufficient to handle the noontime crowds.
Merchandise	A high proportion of souvenir purchases will be for high-margin cloth items such as T-shirts and hats.	Euro Disney guests purchased a much lower proportion of high-margin items than expected.	Europeans preferred low-margin printed souvenirs such as postcards and bumper stickers.

equally likely or to "average out" divergent assumptions into a most likely case. As introduced in Chapter One, planning assumptions must recognize varying levels of uncertainty and differentiate between clear trends, unknowns that are knowable, and residual uncertainty. A framework for classifying planning assumptions based on uncertainty is discussed later in this chapter.

The Importance of Planning Assumptions

Once articulated, planning assumptions allow connectivity in the strategic planning process, establish a common foundation for all who participate in strategy development, and identify critical success factors for the future. In addition, the process of developing planning assumptions is valuable in itself.

Allowing Connectivity in the Planning Process

As noted earlier, there are no facts about the future. Planning assumptions are valuable because they help to connect information from the environmental assessment to specific directions and strategies for the future. By making these connections, planning assumptions ensure that the environmental assessment is a primary input in the strategic planning process. All too often, organizations put aside the environmental assessment while proceeding with what they believe to be the real work of strategic planning: developing future direction and strategies. In doing so, they not only negate the hard work associated with developing the environmental assessment but also frequently ignore information that can be critical to future success. Planning assumptions essentially serve as a reality check in the planning process, forcing the organization to test the wisdom of proposed strategies against informed guesses about the future.

Establishing a Common Foundation

In a typical strategic planning process, members of the planning committee receive the same informational foundation, the envi-

ronmental assessment. Yet even when building from the same platform they often reach differing conclusions about implications for
the future. These differences of opinion must be explored before
proceeding with the development of direction and strategies. Planning assumptions force planning participants to explicitly consider
their own assumptions about the future, and to work together to
identify shared expectations as well as differences of opinion. In
general, once shared expectations are identified, they require little
additional analysis or discussion. Differences of opinion, on the
other hand, help to identify major areas of uncertainty, providing
advance warning that there may be disagreements regarding the
most appropriate strategies to be pursued and highlighting the need
for additional analysis, further discussion, or changes to the planning process.

Articulating Implications for Organizational Success

A set of planning assumptions is not complete unless it includes
implications for the organization's success. In fact, it often is useful
to organize planning assumptions into two categories: assumptions
about the future environment and the associated critical success factors for the future. Table 4.2 shows several specific examples of such
two-part planning assumptions. Implications for success complete
the planning assumptions by answering the question, What does
this likely future trend mean for our organization and its future success? This is a critical step. Without identifying the specific implications of their expectations for the future, organizations risk having
their planning assumptions interpreted differently by various individuals, a hazardous approach when seeking consensus around future
direction and strategies.

Organizational culture greatly influences development of planning assumptions. Conversely, planning assumptions offer signs of
the underlying culture. Consider two health systems that identified
the growth of alternative medicine as a clear environmental trend.
The first system made the assumption that the growing popularity

Table 4.2. Two-Part Planning Assumptions.

Assumptions About the Future Environment ⟹	Implications for Success
The number of people enrolled in managed care plans will continue to grow, from 35 percent of our service area population in 1999 to 45 percent in 2004.	Medical management will be the key to controlling costs.
Care—not just prices—will be more aggressively managed.	New, more effective models will be needed for aligning incentives with private physician groups.
Continued financial pressure will lead to continued consolidation of physicians into larger groups.	
Organized physician groups will increasingly compete with hospitals and health systems for outpatient business.	

of alternative medicine represented an opportunity for its organization. The system understood that to be successful in the future, it would need to prudently assess and pursue investment in selected forms of alternative medicine. The second system, not prone to openness to new approaches, interpreted the expected boom in alternative medicine as a threat, since it would mean that traditional providers would face new types of competition and would be forced to defend their own approaches to healing.

A second example comes from one of six hospitals serving a major metropolitan area with a rapidly growing suburban market.

With a market share of 15 percent in the suburban market, the hospital had always ranked well behind the market leader, whose own market share was 35 percent. To support the hospital's strategic planning process, the vice president of business development drafted planning assumptions for review by the planning committee. One of the assumptions—that the current market leader held an unassailable number-one position in the rapidly growing suburban area—drew strong objections from many members of the planning committee. They felt it was inappropriate to highlight a reality that was unflattering to the organization. In this clash, the hospital's tendency to dismiss its own shortcomings prevailed. Instead of an assumption that reflected the strength of the traditional market leader and an implication that the hospital should seek to position itself as a strong second in the target market, a much more generic assumption that the hospital has "substantial opportunity to enhance its market position" in the suburbs was used.

Benefits of the Process of Developing Planning Assumptions

The process of developing planning assumptions is valuable in itself. A well-designed process elicits active involvement of both resident experts (such as physicians who have testified before the state committee on Medicaid payment rates or a board member who is a renowned economist) and other key constituencies. Early involvement promotes buy-in to the strategic plan. Individuals who trust that the foundation—the environmental assessment and resulting planning assumptions—has been constructed well are much more inclined to support the future direction and strategies.

Another essential outcome is identifying true uncertainties, which requires an iterative process, as was true in developing the environmental assessment. During a first pass at developing planning assumptions, the organization groups aspects of the future environment into two categories: clear trends, for which planning assumptions can be developed, and key uncertainties, for which assumptions cannot be developed, at least based on available information. The organization must then consider whether additional research will help to resolve any uncertainties, turning them into clear trends for which planning assumptions can be articulated. After the required research is completed, the only remaining uncertainties are true, or residual, uncertainties.

A simple example helps to illustrate the value of an iterative process to develop planning assumptions. A staff-model managed care plan investigated the possibility of developing additional satellite physician offices to augment its central medical center, which offered a broad array of full-time primary and specialty physician services. The satellite offices would include full-time primary care physicians, although key specialists would be available at each site only one day each week.

Relying on recent enrollment information, the individuals charged with planning for the satellites agreed that the outlying suburbs would account for substantial new membership growth in the future, a clear trend based on historical information. However, they were divided in their opinions regarding the future importance of providing physician care "close to home" for members. Half of the planners assumed that geographic access to physician services was key to member satisfaction. The others were convinced that members strongly preferred one-stop shopping and would trade off short travel times to their doctor's office in exchange for having all their health needs met at a single site.

To address this impasse in assumptions, the health plan commissioned targeted focus group research. Using the results from the market research, the planning group reached a consensus that enrollees would not significantly value the satellite sites unless a broad range of physician services was offered there full-time. The planners were able to transform an unknown that is knowable into a clear trend, moving the planning process forward.

In the case of the health plan, certain differences of opinion about the future were resolved through additional research. Unfortunately, not all uncertainties can be researched away. For some aspects of the future environment, several alternative futures may seem plausible even after extensive analysis or research. These aspects of the future represent residual uncertainties. In our prior example, a key residual uncertainty was the likely future move on the part of competing health plans. For this aspect of the future, it was impossible to develop a single planning assumption. Instead, **decision analysis** was used to evaluate the appropriateness of the proposed satellite strategy under two fundamentally different potential competitor scenarios: (1) major competitors continue to centralize services at hub medical centers, and (2) major competitors pursue a distributed services approach. Chapter Five presents a discussion of decision analysis, along with other planning tools to address residual uncertainty.

Characteristics of Good Planning Assumptions

Strategic plans are often called road maps for the future. But they are road maps that must be developed before the territory to be navigated is fully charted. Through its planning assumptions, the organization is seeking to paint one or more pictures of the evolving future in which it will operate, thus increasing the likelihood of selecting the right strategic direction and strategies.

Planning assumptions should not address every aspect of the future environment. The key to developing good planning assumptions is to ask the question, What environmental forces will be major market drivers, ultimately having the greatest impact on our future success or failure? By answering this question, the organization identifies the topic areas to be covered in the planning assumptions. Remember: it is just as dangerous to have too many planning assumptions as it is to have too few. Although a sparse set of planning assumptions may paint an incomplete picture of the future, an overly dense set creates confusion about the environmental forces that are most important to understand and monitor over time.

Table 4.3 summarizes the primary market drivers for the health care industry and the associated topic areas for which planning assumptions may be developed. Of course, each organization must

Table 4.3. Market Drivers and Topic Areas.

Market Drivers	Topic Areas
Demographics	Changes in population size and age composition Changes in socioeconomic status Health status
Market demand	Inpatient and outpatient use rates Trends in demand for specific services (outpatient surgery, alternative medicine, etc.)
Industry structure	Consolidation of payers and providers Organization of physicians Presence and growth of niche providers or alternative medicine providers Hospital-physician linkages
Purchasers	Managed care penetration Profitability of managed care plans Preferred payment mechanisms and incentives Contracting criteria Predominance of exclusive contracting Demand for outcomes and other quality measurements
Public policy	Mandated managed care for Medicaid enrollees Impact of a patient's bill of rights Changes to the Medicare payment system
Consumer expectations and behaviors	Provider selection criteria Demand for alternative medicine Access to information Degree of participation in health care decisions
Competitor strategies	Merger, affiliation, or integration strategies Ambulatory network development Physician strategies Cost, quality, and customer service
Product innovation and technological change	Clinical breakthroughs Technological advances

take into account its own unique challenges and circumstances, tailoring its planning assumptions accordingly.

Good planning assumptions do not simply focus on key market drivers; they share several other characteristics:

- They incorporate measurable information, whenever possible. Planning assumptions that include measurable information articulate expectations regarding the likely degree, as well as direction, of change. The more specific a planning assumption is, the easier it is for planning participants to understand the magnitude of response required for success. For example, a planning assumption stated as "a higher proportion of hospital surgeries will be performed on an outpatient basis" is difficult to interpret. In comparison, an assumption that "by 2005, three-quarters of all hospital surgeries will be performed on an outpatient basis" invites specific strategic responses.

- Good assumptions facilitate effective monitoring. Based on a planning assumption that the proportion of hospital surgeries performed on an outpatient basis has peaked at 65 percent, a hospital might decide not to invest in upgrading its outpatient surgical facilities. It might also decide that, should the proportion reach 70 percent, it will reexamine the need for such an upgrade. Unless measurable information is included in the planning assumptions, it is difficult to use them as triggers for rethinking or modifying strategies.

- Good planning assumptions clearly articulate the pressure for change, serving as the rationale for an organization's strategic intent and strategies. If individuals across the organization do not understand the need for change, they are unlikely to support the change being recommended. Planning assumptions must be clear enough that individuals not participating in the planning process can understand why particular strategies are being pursued and others are not. Clarity of planning assumptions is critical to generating support and enthusiasm for the strategic plan.

As noted earlier, good planning assumptions identify not only how the environment will change but what the external change means for the organization's own future success. Although a single planning assumption may have its own implications for success, most implications are identified by considering the interactions among several planning assumptions. Often but not always, implications for success fall into one of these categories: image and reputation, organizational culture, scope and geographic distribution of services, relationships with physicians, quality and customer service, cost position, participation in teaching and research, and positioning as an employer.

Developing Planning Assumptions

Thus far in this chapter, we have explored the theory behind planning assumptions. We turn our focus next to the practice of developing them.

Key findings from the environmental assessment should serve as the basis for specific planning assumptions. Difficulty in translating the results of the environmental assessment into future assumptions is a good indicator that your assessment either focuses on the wrong analyses or is incomplete. An example of translating the information from the environmental assessment into planning assumptions is in Table 4.4. Note that the planning assumptions include assumptions about both the future environment and the associated critical success factors.

How can planning assumptions with measurable information be developed? Although there are numerous methods in theory, three practical approaches have stood the test of time in health care strategy formulation: the "issues questionnaire," the Delphi forecasting method, and quantitative forecasting techniques.

The Issues Questionnaire

An **issues questionnaire** is a process facilitation tool to elicit input from key individuals regarding their own expectations for the future. Administered as a written survey, it typically contains a series of

Table 4.4. Translating the Environmental Assessment.

Historical Information $\Longrightarrow$	Assumptions About the Future Environment $\Longrightarrow$	Implications for Success
Over the last five years, inpatient days per 1,000 population have declined at 3 percent per year, while outpatient visits have grown at 4 percent per year.	Over the next five years, inpatient days per 1,000 population will decrease by an additional 15 percent, while outpatient visits will grow 20 percent.	A higher proportion of resources and investment must be targeted for outpatient services.
Historically, operating margins for inpatient services have been significantly higher than for outpatient services.	Changes in demand will substitute historically low-margin services for services which have had much higher margins in the past.	To maintain inpatient volume, the hospital must increase market share in its current market or expand its coverage to new markets.
		Financial performance of outpatient services must be improved.

questions about specific aspects of the future environment. The results of the issues questionnaire are used as the starting point for developing assumptions about the future. There are three specific advantages of the issues questionnaire approach:

1. The issues questionnaire forces all planning participants to explicitly examine their own assumptions about the future. Without an issues questionnaire or other similar tool, planning assumptions may be developed according to group politics rather than the best thinking of the overall planning group.

2. Because it is confidential, the issues questionnaire is a forum for individuals to express unpopular or dissenting opinions. In an era of uncertainty, it is especially important for the organization to be open to nontraditional thinking. Properly structured, an issues questionnaire can stimulate such creative thinking.

3. The issues questionnaire is an effective tool for obtaining input from a large number of individuals, including both resident experts and individuals who may not otherwise participate in the planning process. Results of the issues questionnaire can be cross-tabulated based on any number of demographic factors, allowing easy comparison of the perspectives of various constituency groups.

A word of caution: the issues questionnaire is not a substitute for the environmental assessment. It is a tool for building on the results of the environmental assessment to articulate expectations for the future. In our experience, the issues questionnaire tends to work best when combined with group discussion. It is through discussion that planning participants explore the reasons for their responses, often discovering that their views are either farther apart or closer together than written results, on their own, would suggest. Exhibit 4.1 offers an example of a question from an issues questionnaire used with a health system's affiliated specialists. The majority response to this question suggests a planning assumption, which in turn implies critical success factors for the system.

Poorly structured issues questionnaires can complicate rather than facilitate development of planning assumptions. When structuring the issues questionnaire, it is important to:

- Emphasize that there are no right or wrong answers. Remember: there are no facts about the future. The real value of the issues questionnaire lies in its ability to foster discussion among individuals with diverse opinions.

- Stress and maintain confidentiality. Creative thinking is most likely to occur under these circumstances.

- Include the full range of potential responses for each question, including options that are plausible but not popular.

Exhibit 4.1. Translating the Issues Questionnaire.

Question:

Which of the following statements best describes your assessment of the supply of primary care physicians in the service area?

    A. Oversupply: there are too many primary care physicians.

    B. Undersupply: there are too few primary care physicians.

    C. Just right: there is an appropriate and adequate supply of primary care physicians.

Responses:

    A. 15 percent

    B. 70 percent

    C. 15 percent

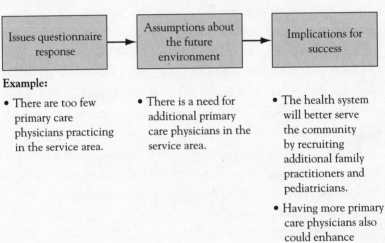

Example:

Issues questionnaire response	Assumptions about the future environment	Implications for success
• There are too few primary care physicians practicing in the service area.	• There is a need for additional primary care physicians in the service area.	• The health system will better serve the community by recruiting additional family practitioners and pediatricians. • Having more primary care physicians also could enhance affiliated specialists' satisfaction with the health system.

- Word each question in a way that is easy to answer and tabulate. Multiple choice questions usually work best.

- Keep it short. Questionnaires that can be completed in ten to fifteen minutes typically have a higher return rate than longer, more complicated surveys. Having a time limit means that the questionnaire must focus on the most critical future issues for the organization.

Delphi Forecasting

Delphi forecasting is a second approach to developing planning assumptions. The term is derived from the oracle at Delphi, a shrine to the Greek god Apollo where pilgrims traveled in search of advice on both personal matters and affairs of the state. Like an issues questionnaire, the Delphi forecasting method uses a series of questions to which panelists respond individually and anonymously. After each question is answered, the panelists are given all individual responses and encouraged to comment on their own responses as well as the combined panel results.

Following group discussion, the panelists submit revised answers to the same set of questions. The iterative Delphi forecasting process reduces the effects of personal agenda or bias and supplies a wealth of information that contributes to overall understanding of the future health care environment.

The Society for Healthcare Strategy and Market Development has recently developed a publication using Delphi forecasting to predict health care industry trends. Titled *Beyond 2000: Health Care Trends in the New Millennium,* the study addresses a broad range of industry trends, including the health care economy, federal and state health reform, the role of managed care, consumer and purchaser behavior, industry consolidation, and physician practice and compensation structures. The study is an excellent resource for health care organizations as they develop planning assumptions (Coile, 1999).

Forecasting Techniques

Planning assumptions can also be developed using basic quantitative forecasting techniques. Forecasting is a method for predicting the future in accordance with historical trends. Two things are required to develop an appropriate and reasonable forecast: an understanding or estimate of the current position of the variable, and an assumption regarding the expected change in the variable.

In developing quantitative forecasts, many health care organizations underestimate the time and energy required to accurately assess the current position of the variable. In general, organizations should spend as much time determining current position as they spend forecasting future change (Webber and Peters, 1983). The majority of forecasting errors are a result of failure to define the current status or starting point. Attempts to quantify the supply of physicians in a particular market are a case in point. Because it is difficult to pinpoint exactly how many physicians are practicing in a given market at any given time, it is especially difficult to develop assumptions about their numbers in the future.

The second step in developing any forecast is to identify the factors that can contribute to changes in the variable. This step is particularly challenging in a rapidly transforming industry such as health care, since the forces likely to have the biggest impact may be most difficult to predict. As discussed in Chapter One, technological or pharmaceutical breakthroughs could fundamentally alter demand for specific health care services. But we do not yet have the information to fully understand their potential impact.

In an era of uncertainty, forecasting based on historical trends carries certain risks. In particular, it can also unduly anchor thinking to old trends and realities. Managers often fail to consider radical changes, however unlikely or improbable, that would significantly alter their markets (Porter, 1985). In 1962, an executive with Decca Recording declined to offer the Beatles a record contract, asserting that "We don't like their sound. Groups of guitars are on the way out" (Shoemaker, 1995, p. 26). It is important to avoid overreliance on historical truths; they always are subject to major market changes.

Conclusion

Because they are tools for envisioning the future, planning assumptions are essential to strategic planning in an era of uncertainty. Through the process of developing planning assumptions, the organization is able to articulate shared expectations for the future, explicitly acknowledge varying degrees of future uncertainty, and isolate key environmental factors that may be of critical importance to future success but for which no single planning assumption can be developed. Planning assumptions also can serve as a starting point for valuable monitoring. If developed correctly, they highlight key aspects of the environment to be monitored over time to ensure early warning of major environmental changes and challenges. Planning assumptions are the foundation for direction and strategies. It should be as unthinkable to develop a strategic plan without planning assumptions as it would be to erect a bridge without its pilings.

Lessons Learned

✓ Planning assumptions have been used in health care for many years, but new approaches to developing them are needed to address the reality of uncertainty about the future.

✓ Planning assumptions help a health care organization anticipate its future environment, contemplating potential challenges and opportunities as well as future requirements for organizational success.

✓ Good planning assumptions focus on key market forces, incorporate measurable information, and articulate the pressures for change.

✓ The process of developing planning assumptions is itself valu-able, helping to build early support for the strategic plan and to dif-ferentiate among clear future trends, unknowns that are knowable, and residual uncertainties.

✓ Planning assumptions connect the environmental assessment to strategic intent and strategies. If it is difficult to translate the results of the environmental assessment into planning assumptions, it is likely that your assessment focuses on the wrong things or is incomplete.

✓ Issues questionnaires, Delphi forecasting, and quantitative forecasting are facilitation tools for moving from the environmental assessment to development of specific assumptions about the future.

✓ Organizational culture greatly influences development of planning assumptions.

5

. . . .

Tools to Address Uncertainty

Marian C. Jennings, Scott B. Clay, and Erin P. Carr

In an era of uncertainty, how can organizational leaders synthesize a broad range of uncertainties into a manageable framework for formulating strategy? What changes in traditional planning tools does this require? This chapter introduces three of the most effective tools for addressing uncertainty: scenario planning, decision analysis, and game theory. As seen in the References and Suggested Reading, a large body of literature on these subjects, both practical and theoretical, is available. However, this chapter focuses on the practical application of these tools for health care providers, using theory only to introduce principles.

The new planning tools discussed in this chapter are not used simultaneously; each is appropriate in its own situation. However, they do contain similar elements and concepts because they all have the common goal of identifying and understanding the impact of uncertainty. Recognizing that there is no crystal ball that gives a clear vision of the future, leaders can use these tools to develop a shared mental picture of the elements that potential futures may include.

As discussed in Chapter Two, scenario planning, decision analysis, and game theory complement rather than replace other components of the strategic planning process (the environmental assessment, planning assumptions, goals and strategies, and financial planning). Although the new planning tools described in this chapter are not sufficient alone to determine an organization's strategy, they constitute a structured framework for understanding the uncertainties inherent in the future.

Scenario Planning

Scenario planning was originally developed in the 1950s by the Rand Corporation for the U.S. government to study how nuclear wars might start. The government needed a way to understand, and prepare for, the myriad possibilities that could spark a catastrophic event. The government found scenario planning to be so useful that it continues to use Rand scenarios today. For example, one of Rand's current high-profile scenarios is a compelling story of how a nuclear war between India and Pakistan begins by the year 2006 ("Think Tank Predicts . . . ," 1999).

Royal Dutch/Shell is widely credited with pioneering use of scenario planning for strategy in the business community. In the late 1970s, scenario planning helped the company to prepare for a drop in oil prices, while conventional wisdom in the industry predicted continuing high prices. Based on this "possible future," Shell decided not to buy expensive oil reserves. When the Middle East oil cartel dissolved and Russian oil reserves became available to the west, oil prices dropped and, unlike most of its competitors, Shell was able to take advantage of the lower prices (Hudson, 1995).

More recently, scenario planning has emerged as a widely used tool in a variety of industries. Rapidly changing industries such as biotechnology have embraced scenario planning to anticipate the impact of uncertainties including consumer sentiment and government regulation. Industry giants Monsanto, Hoechst, Du Pont, Eli Lilly, Novartis, and others have banded together to sponsor ten-year and thirty-year scenario development projects (Feder, 1999). Other sectors, from energy and transportation to electronics and education, are also using scenario planning to "practice the future."

Scenario Planning in Health Care

Although infrequently used in health care, scenario planning is not entirely new to the industry. In 1991, the Healthcare Forum Foundation Leadership Center developed five scenarios for their national study "Bridging the Leadership Gap in Healthcare" (Bezold, 1992):

1. Continued growth/high-tech: providers predict and manage illness earlier and more successfully through continuing advances in expensive biomedical technology. Healthcare expenditures continue to grow as a percentage of GNP.

2. Hard times/government leadership: the United States adopts a Canadian-style national health insurance system, and two systems of health care emerge as one-third of Americans buy gap insurance.

3. Buyer's market: market competition leads to better, less expensive service, but better social policies blunt the inequities of the stronger market approach.

4. A new civilization/healing and health care: the focus of health care broadens from the individual to the community and the environment as health care organizations merge with other community organizations.

5. Healing and health care: alternative therapies increase, and the role of spirit in health care leads to greater focus on "healing."

These scenarios, developed by the Institute for Alternative Futures, were used to identify the values and competencies that will be most important for health care leaders in the twenty-first century.

Similarly in 1997, the American Hospital Association, with the assistance of Northeast Consulting Resources, developed scenarios for the health care industry. The AHA scenarios were built around these provider models, to stimulate thinking about divergent models of health care delivery:

- Branded care: a few for-profit, branded national health care companies control over half of the inpatient and outpatient capacity of the U.S. health care system.

- Best care: insurer-based organizations take advantage of information-based health care and emerge as integrators of services.

- Extender care: leading primary care groups improve quality, lower cost, and gain an increasing percentage of primary care and outpatient volume through aggressive use of physician extenders.

- Surgicare: for-profit chain of surgery-centered facilities competes head-to-head with hospitals by focusing its resources on a single core business.

- Pathway, Inc.: disease management companies market themselves to payers as lower-cost, effective providers for certain chronic and life-threatening conditions.

The Healthcare Forum and AHA projects were industrywide in scope, but other leading health care providers, such as Allina Health System, Kaiser Permanente, Sutter Health Care, and M. D. Anderson Cancer Center all have used scenario-based planning to help develop strategies for their specific circumstances.

The Scenario Planning Tool

Scenario planning is a systematic approach for imagining alternative futures, each of which is plausible but not assured. This tool is used to identify potential risks and alternative environments. Scenario planning helps to simplify complex interactions and synthesize large amounts of data into a limited number of possible future states to help leaders overcome "analysis paralysis" and focus on key issues.

Each scenario tells a story about how the future might unfold and how critical elements might interact. For example, the Health-care Forum's hard-times/government-leadership scenario describes the interaction of health care economic factors, societal expectations for health care, and government responses under a particular set of circumstances.

By developing various scenarios, leaders can "practice the future" by considering the series of events that lead to each future and the options they would have for establishing the organization's strategic position or influencing key events. Leaders also can identify **trigger points** for each scenario (indicators that the market is moving toward or away from a specific direction) to monitor key events as the future unfolds. These trigger points can serve as important signals for adjusting strategy as necessary.

For example, clear trigger points that the AHA's branded-care scenario was not evolving include the government's investigation of Columbia Healthcare, Columbia's subsequent change in leadership, and the resulting shift in corporate strategy from aggressive growth to mending fences. During the mid-1990s, the conventional wisdom was that Columbia would continue its aggressive growth, and among its competitors many strategies focused on "defense against Columbia." If more providers had anticipated Columbia's reversal, they would have been better prepared for today's reality. Incidentally, the final chapter on Columbia (now HCA) and other large for-profit systems has not yet been written. It is still uncertain.

Scenario planning is designed to broaden the perspective of leaders, not to predict the future with certainty. The process of scenario planning is useful in that it helps leaders consider a broad range of possibilities that are plausible but not necessarily in line with today's conventional wisdom. Although scenario planning is useful for identifying uncertainties and exploring alternative environments, it is only a tool, not a final outcome such as a vision or strategic plan.

As indicated by the Healthcare Forum and AHA examples, scenarios are distinct—and frequently extreme—representations about how the future might unfold. Often, they are not mutually exclusive. In fact, the real future is likely to contain selected elements of various scenarios. In the AHA example, it is quite possible for extender-care and surgicare models to coexist.

Why is it important to consider alternative futures before developing your organization's strategic intent? Many of history's greatest experts have relied with certainty upon grossly inaccurate predictions. Apart from examples in earlier chapters, here is another. In 1977, the president of Digital Equipment commented that "there is no reason for any individual to have a computer in their home." Can we be sure that our current experts' forecasts are any more reliable? It may be as difficult today for a hospital CEO to anticipate the impact of the human genome project on health care delivery as it was for the president of DEC to see a need for home computers in 1977.

When to Use Scenario Planning

Scenario planning is most useful when levels of uncertainty are high for several critically important assumptions, such as governmental regulation or reform initiatives, consolidation of competitors in the local market, or the long-term effect of "managed care backlash." Specifically, scenario planning is appropriate when an organization recognizes that it faces a broad range of possible futures that cannot be easily segregated into discrete alternate futures (see Chapter One for full discussion of levels of uncertainty).

Paul J. H. Shoemaker, a leading figure in scenario planning, provides guidance (1995) on the conditions under which an organization benefits especially from scenario planning:

- Too many costly surprises have occurred in the past.

- The organization does not identify or generate new opportunities.

- The quality of current strategic thinking is low (for example, focus on cost containment but not strategic partnerships, innovative delivery alternatives, or new services).

- The organization wants a common framework for thinking about the future without stifling diversity.

- Competitors are using scenario planning.

Even if scenario planning seems appropriate for all these reasons, it is effective only in organizations in which the CEO understands and supports this approach. Scenario planning requires willingness to suspend commonly held beliefs about the future—the ability to say "I really don't know how the future will unfold." Some leaders are uncomfortable acknowledging their inability to predict the future and consequently are unable to truly participate in or benefit from scenario building.

Process for Developing Scenarios

Many industrywide scenario planning processes, such as the Health-care Forum and AHA examples, involve extensive participation and are time-consuming. Individual hospitals and health systems need a practical approach to scenario planning that fits into the overall strategic planning process and addresses organization-specific issues. The practical eight-step scenario planning process that we describe here builds on the findings from the environmental assessment (Chapter Three) and planning assumptions (Chapter Four) and allows leaders to develop organization-specific scenarios that improve their ability to establish strategic intent.

Step One: Define the Scope of Scenario Development

The first step in scenario development is to state explicitly the purpose or goals of the exercise. In this book, we assume that scenario planning is being used to help answer the fundamental strategic question(s) facing the organization. However, this tool also may be used for objectives more limited in scope. For example, the M. D. Anderson Cancer Center at the University of Texas used scenario planning to develop a ten-year capital plan for its 4.5 million square feet of facilities (Ingalls, 1999). With the initial purpose targeted on facilities development, the composition of the planning team and the range of issues were clearly focused.

Once the overall purpose or scope has been identified, leaders must identify the time frame for the scenarios. Many industrywide scenario planning exercises look ten to twenty years into the future to identify very-long-range issues. However, for most individual hospitals and health systems, a planning horizon of five years is practical. There are cases in which looking out ten or more years is useful, especially if the fundamental strategic question is likely to involve large, long-term capital commitments (such as a replacement hospital with a thirty-year useful life).

Step Two: Identify Major Stakeholders

It is important to involve key stakeholders actively in scenario planning. In considering who to involve in the process, it is useful to ask, "Who has an interest in the organization's key issues? Who is affected most by them? Who can influence them?"

In a recent scenario planning exercise, the biotechnology industry invited one of its most outspoken critics to participate. Known in the industry as the "abominable no-man," this outside activist provided a valuable perspective about the future of the industry (Feder, 1999). Similarly for health care providers, although sometimes painful it is important to include those with divergent opinions (such as the "lone ranger" physician who constantly questions conventional wisdom).

Step Three: Questions to the Clairvoyant

In our experience, the simple planning exercise Questions to the Clairvoyant (mentioned in Chapter Three) has proven to be an effective and practical tool to quickly identify the core issues for scenario development. Here is how to conduct this exercise.

First, ask participants to answer the question, "If you could pose only three questions to a clairvoyant, somebody who could actually foretell the future of this organization and its environment in five years, what questions would you ask?"

A useful warm-up exercise is to ask participants to look back and think about what they wish they had known about today's environment five or ten years ago. This gives participants a frame of reference about the potential magnitude and impact of unexpected changes. For example, five years ago, most health care executives would have liked to know the answers to questions such as "Will capitation become the dominant form of payment in five years?" or "Will a few large integrated delivery systems, with large, owned primary care components, dominate our market?"

Second, after all participants have identified their questions, ask them each to answer their own questions in two ways:

1. "Imagine the future is a good one, rolling out as you hope it will. How would you as a clairvoyant answer your own three questions?"

2. "Imagine the future is a bad one, rolling out as you dread it may. How would you as a clairvoyant answer your own three questions?"

Step Four: Identify Themes, Trends, and Uncertainties

The Questions to the Clairvoyant exercise generates a long list of uncertainties and predicted outcomes that are directly relevant to the organization. If fifteen participants are involved, the exercise can generate as many as forty-five key uncertainties (three per participant). To synthesize the results of the exercise, instruct staff or a small working group to analyze the individual answers for:

• Common themes: although the exercise elicits many answers, the results for most groups are easy to cluster into a few powerful underlying themes, such as "continued struggle for control of the health care premium dollar."

- Clear trends and forces: these are the trends that are expected to play out in all scenarios. Individuals mention them as part of their best-case and worst-case responses. An example is increased competition. In the best case, the organization rises to the competitive challenge or creates obstacles to new competitors entering the market. In the worst case, the organization sees its market position erode as traditional competitors flourish and new competitors enter the market.

- Major uncertainties: these areas of uncertainty have a significant impact on the organization. For example, how active a role consumers play in their health care decision making was a major uncertainty recognized by one specialty hospital located in a metropolitan market.

The common themes are used in the next step to identify the fundamental strategic question for the organization. The clear trends form the basis for any hedge strategies, those that work under any scenario. The major uncertainties determine the scenarios themselves.

Step Five: Identify the Fundamental Strategic Question(s)

Typically, health care organizations have one or two fundamental strategic questions they are trying to answer. Here are examples:

- Can our organization continue to be successful as an independent provider?

- Should we continue to pursue our vision as _____? (fill in the blank)

- Is our mix of services appropriate for the future needs of our community?

Identifying the organization's fundamental strategic question is very important, and often very difficult. To discover the fundamental question, review the common themes from Questions to the Clairvoyant. Also review the results of the environmental assessment, particularly the constituency interviews, which included questions such as "What are the most critical issues facing the organization?" Usually, the fundamental question is a combination of key themes repeated in exercises throughout the planning process.

The fundamental questions are unique to each organization. For example, one hospital, positioned as a specialty provider with high-profile physicians and an excellent reputation, posed the question, "Will patients and physicians value us enough to demand access to our services and ensure that we receive a fair price for our services?" This question emerged because the hospital's historical success was anchored on its ability to draw patients, thanks to its excellent reputation for specific services and its low-cost position.

Step Six: Develop a Scenario Matrix

Among the key uncertainties identified, the planning group needs to choose the two that have the greatest impact on the fundamental strategic question facing the organization. The two key uncertainties form the X and Y axes of a scenario matrix. The four scenarios of the matrix represent combinations of the plausible extremes for the two greatest uncertainties facing the organization.

The example shown in Figure 5.1 is based upon the fundamental question discussed in step five: "Will patients and physicians value us enough to demand access to our services and ensure we receive a fair price for our services?" Since the answer to this question relies heavily on the role of consumers and the structure of its competitive market, the hospital in this example identified (1) the degree of consumer activism and (2) regional system consolidation as the most important areas of uncertainty.

Once the uncertainties on the X and Y axes have been chosen, name the four quadrants. Carefully consider names for the scenarios. They are much easier to understand and remember if the

Figure 5.1. Example of Future Health Care Environment in Our Market.

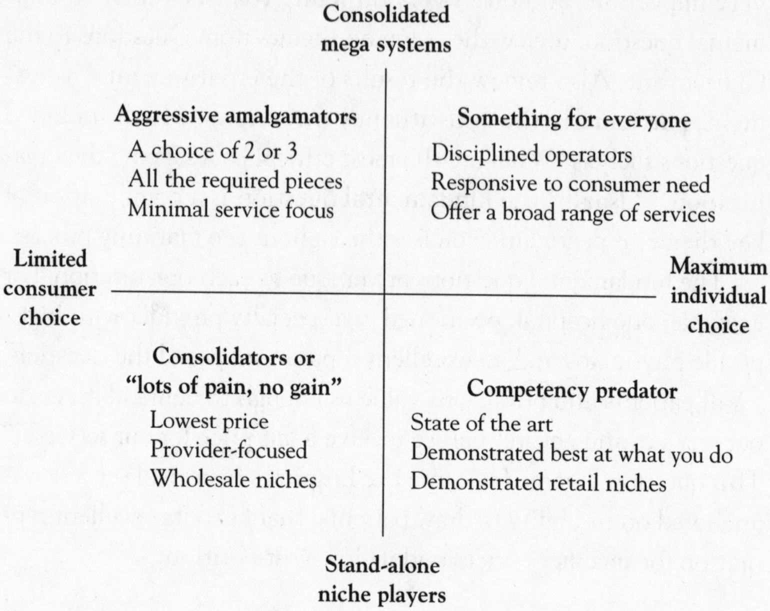

**Consolidated
mega systems**

Aggressive amalgamators	**Something for everyone**
A choice of 2 or 3	Disciplined operators
All the required pieces	Responsive to consumer need
Minimal service focus	Offer a broad range of services

**Limited
consumer
choice** ———————————————————— **Maximum
individual
choice**

| **Consolidators or
"lots of pain, no gain"**	**Competency predator**
Lowest price	State of the art
Provider-focused	Demonstrated best at what you do
Wholesale niches	Demonstrated retail niches

**Stand-alone
niche players**

Highest uncertainties

- Passive versus active consumer (X)
- Structure of industry (Y)

essence of the major theme is captured in the title. For example, the names of the AHA's branded-care and Pathway, Inc., scenarios concisely summarize the main themes.

Next, flesh out the scenarios by developing core descriptions or themes for each quadrant and organizing possible outcomes and trends around them. In describing the skeleton scenarios, refer back to the key trends and themes identified in step four. Most of the major trends or themes should be addressed in each scenario. For example, the full text of the Healthcare Forum scenarios (Bezold, 1992) describes the roles of providers, health care expenditures, government policy, and biomedical technology.

After developing the scenario themes, check them for relevance, consistency, and plausibility. Shoemaker (1995) suggests three tests of internal consistency. First, are the scenarios compatible with the chosen time frame? Second, do the scenarios combine outcomes of uncertainties that go together, such as low medical inflation and a continued trend toward open-access managed care products? Third, are major stakeholders placed in positions they do not like but can change?

Step Seven: Clarify How Each Quadrant Is Likely to Affect the Organization

In anticipating the impact each scenario will have on the organization, first identify the degree of change each one represents for the organization. Is it consistent with the organization's current vision and priorities, or does it challenge current thinking? Second, what risks does each scenario present for the organization? In assessing the risks and opportunities inherent in each scenario, it is helpful to address key questions:

- What do we need to do to "win" in each quadrant?

- How does our strategic question play out in each quadrant?

- What does it make sense to do across all scenarios?

- If we select one quadrant as our preferred positioning and the market evolves otherwise, can we recover?

Step Eight: Establish Trigger Points for Monitoring

Finally, identify for each quadrant key events that lead to the endpoint scenario. For example, key events that lead to "competency predator" in Figure 5.1 include:

- Medical inflation remaining low

- Open-access HMOs eclipsing traditional HMOs in number of enrollees

- Capitation for hospital payments virtually disappearing

- Consumers demonstrating willingness to accept increasing copays to get the best

- Loose-knit health system alliances unraveling and merger-and-acquisition activity slowing

- Focused-factory hospital chains, such as MedCath, growing in number and strength

Step eight is useful for several reasons. First, it builds the scenarios into realistic stories that develop over time. Second, it helps to test plausibility by offering a series of milestones that lead logically to the end point. Finally, it allows the organization to establish early-warning signals about which direction critical environmental factors are going.

Evaluating the Scenarios

Once the scenarios have been developed, use these criteria to evaluate their quality and appropriateness:

- Do they address the fundamental strategic question(s) facing your organization?

- Are they recognizable and consistent with the thought processes of the decision makers?

- Does each present a plausible future?

- Do they represent fundamentally different futures rather than variations on a single theme?

- Do they challenge conventional wisdom?

- Does each describe an equilibrium or stable state of affairs?

Benefits and Drawbacks of Scenario Planning

When leaders in organizations face high levels of uncertainty, they typically react in one of three ways: (1) they focus exclusively on one prediction of the future (conventional wisdom), (2) they disagree internally about the future and agree that several options have merit, or (3) they are immobilized by the degree of uncertainty in the environment and consider planning to be worthless.

Scenario planning helps leaders organize complex uncertainties into manageable "snapshots" of the future so they can minimize these typical reactions. One of the primary benefits of scenario planning is that it encourages decision makers to consider possibilities they fear or will otherwise ignore. It is an approach that challenges conventional wisdom and increases tolerance for ambiguity. This tool also allows participants to synthesize large amounts of information into a limited number of stories that are easy to grasp intuitively. Finally, scenario planning is able to incorporate complex elements that cannot be formally modeled, such as government regulation, societal value shifts, and innovations. For these reasons, scenario planning is particularly useful in helping leaders understand the range of possibilities facing them, and in dispelling the belief that much of the uncertainty they face is unknowable.

Scenario planning is a useful tool for planning under uncertainty, but it is frequently used inappropriately. Two common mistakes are believing that scenarios are predictions of the future rather than tools for broadening perspectives, and treating them as being informational rather than as a tool for participatory learning.

Although scenario planning is a valuable new tool in the strategic planning toolkit, it adds value only by facilitating strategic thinking. Like any other tool, it is affected by the biases of the participants and dependent upon the skill of its facilitators. Although scenario planning is designed to help organizations understand uncertainty, it does not resolve it. No one scenario is likely to contain all elements of the real future, but even so scenario planning is often misused as a predictive tool.

Decision Analysis

Scenario planning deals with a wide range of uncertainties; decision analysis is most effective if there are a discrete number of alternatives to be considered. By clearly linking decisions with their probable outcomes, decision analysis permits a structured approach to mapping the future consequences of decisions.

History and Applications of Decision Analysis

Decision analysis, as we know it today, has been applied extensively for the last forty years. It evolved from operations research, game theory, and the study of behaviorism in the 1950s. Its application to business strategy has been successful because decision analysis gives an organization a road map outlining the decision-making process. This chapter focuses on practical application of this road map—the decision tree, which is a graphic representation of the decision-outcome pathways.

Decision analysis has been used in investigating murders, assessing workforce requirements, and determining moves in chess. In health care, decision analysis is being used with increasing frequency in health policy planning, clinical information and decision-support systems, and in developing clinical protocols. Decision analysis allows physicians to integrate evidence-based medicine with patient preferences (Lilford, Parker, Braunholtz, and Chard, 1998). Furthermore, it has become a very useful tool for health economists and managers. In the decision analysis framework, quality and costs of health care decisions can be evaluated concurrently (Brasel and Weigelt, 1997).

Decision Analysis Basics

Decisions are needed in situations where two or more courses of action are available and only one action can be taken. Decision analysis is useful in determining the best strategy when a decision maker is faced with several discrete alternatives in an uncertain future. It promotes forward thinking and forces organizations to contemplate potential paths of change within the industry.

The decision analysis framework helps to identify the likely winners and losers in alternative situations; perhaps more important, it helps to quantify what is at stake for companies that follow status quo strategies. Such analysis is often the key to making the case for strategic change (Courtney, Kirkland, and Viguerie, 1997). An organized approach to applying decision theory involves five phases.

Phase One: State the Decision Problem

The initial phase in decision analysis is to identify the decision at hand and the available choices. Identifying action steps, decisions to be made, and possible outcomes is also part of stating the decision problem. All outcomes should be mutually exclusive. When structuring the decision problem, sunk costs and decisions that have already been made should be excluded from the decision-making process. For example, people often finish their meal at a restaurant not because they are hungry but rather because they don't want to be wasteful. However, the cost of the meal becomes a sunk cost as soon as it is ordered, so it should not be a factor when deciding how much to eat. Only future decisions are relevant.

Once the decision process is clearly defined, confirm that the possible outcomes are significant enough to warrant continuing the decision analysis process. Do not waste time on courses of action that cannot be carried out, or problems with outcomes that have inconsequential impact.

For example, a hospital CEO is considering purchasing an additional MRI (the decision problem). The two obvious choices (action steps) are to acquire the MRI or not acquire it. The potential market share outcomes from this decision range from an increase of 20 percent to a decrease of 10 percent. Since the potential outcomes are material, the CEO should proceed with the decision analysis process.

Phase Two: Construct a Decision Tree

A decision tree is a graphic representation of the decision-making process, used to analyze sequential decisions. By following a path on a decision tree, a decision maker easily understands the potential outcomes of a decision. Decision trees are effective in modeling situations with a limited number of decision points and repetition of events.

Decision nodes, chance nodes, and outcomes represent events on the decision tree. A decision node, usually denoted by a square or box (see Figure 5.2), is a point in the decision tree where the decision maker must choose among several alternatives. A chance node, usually symbolized with a circle, is a point in the decision tree where the outcome is uncertain or at risk. At decision nodes, the decision maker has control. At chance branches, the direction of the path on the decision tree cannot be directly controlled by the decision maker. However, the outcome may be influenced in some cases.

Figure 5.2 presents a decision tree for the MRI example. The decision nodes represent the choices between purchasing or not purchasing the MRI and marketing or not marketing it. The other nodes on the tree—a competitor purchasing the MRI, and the impact of marketing on market share—are chance nodes since the decision maker has minimal or no control over these factors. Accurately constructing the decision tree is vital since conclusions that come from flawed decision trees may be at best inaccurate and at worst dangerous (Brasel and Weigelt, 1997).

Phase Three: Accept Uncontrollable Events

The third phase in the decision analysis process is accepting what can and cannot be controlled. If people act, they can fall victim to delusions of control. Chance events are often treated as if they involve skill and are therefore controllable; a clear example is how people often want to pick their lottery numbers instead of having numbers randomly selected. Similarly, in developing provider-sponsored

Figure 5.2. Decision Tree Example: MRI Purchase.

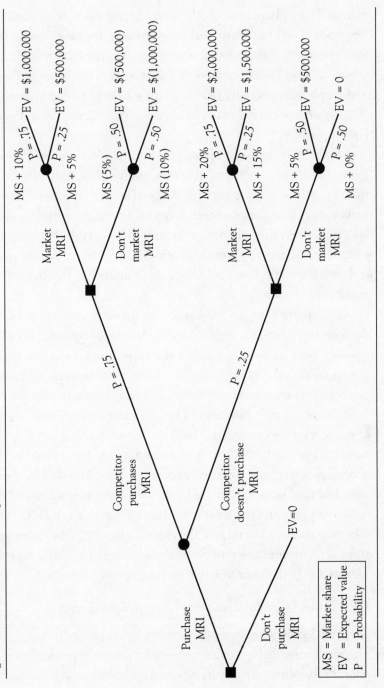

MS + 10% P = .75 EV = $1,000,000
MS + 5%   P = .25 EV = $500,000

MS (5%)   P = .50 EV = $(500,000)
MS (10%) P = .50 EV = $(1,000,000)

MS + 20% P = .75 EV = $2,000,000
MS + 15% P = .25 EV = $1,500,000

MS + 5%   P = .50 EV = $500,000
MS + 0%   P = .50 EV = 0

Market
MRI

Don't
market
MRI

Market
MRI

Don't
market
MRI

P = .75

P = .25

Competitor
purchases
MRI

Competitor
doesn't purchase
MRI

EV=0

Purchase
MRI

Don't
purchase
MRI

MS = Market share
EV = Expected value
P = Probability

managed care plans, many health care executives overestimated the hospital's ability to control utilization to keep medical costs in line with premiums. Tremendous losses owing to such uncontrollable factors as adverse selection, random fluctuation in claims experience, and (most unexpectedly to many) their own physicians' overutilization of services led many health care providers to divest their health plans.

Much of the value in identifying controllable events is distinguishing between a controllable event and uncertainty in a situation. As with scenario planning, decision analysis requires decision makers to acknowledge uncertainty and accept the fact that there are times when they are not in charge. Alternatively, if an organization is paralyzed by uncertainty and does nothing at points where it does have control, or could have some influence, this has consequences of its own.

Continuing with the MRI example, there are two points in the decision tree where the decision maker has direct control. He or she does not have a choice to make at the two chance nodes, but this is not to say that this person cannot influence an outcome. Although the decision maker can control the marketing efforts to promote the MRI, he or she only influences—but does not control—the impact of the marketing campaign. The term *chance node* implies that the outcome is entirely random. A more appropriate term would be *risk node*, since outcomes are usually influenced or controlled by someone. The final outcomes in the MRI example, market share and the resulting profit, are uncertain, but there are actions the CEO can take that increase the odds of the desired outcome. The uncertainties that surround the competitor's purchase of an MRI must be accepted as both uncontrollable and not open to influence.

Phase Four: Assign Probabilities to Uncontrollable Events

Rational decisions are based on assessing future possibilities and likelihoods. These likelihoods are expressed in terms of probabilities, or odds. Probabilities are usually assigned according to both empirical facts and individual beliefs. Therefore, it is very difficult to develop probabilities that are free of bias. Inaccurate assignment of probabilities can lead to misguided decisions. Probabilities drive the expected value calculation and therefore the likely recommendation.

The CEO contemplating the purchase of an MRI estimates a 75 percent chance of the competitor doing the same. This is based on a combination of historical competition, a documented need for an additional MRI in the area, and gut feeling. Likewise, the probability assignments for the impact of marketing encompass both intuition and factual information.

Phase Five: Analyze the Expected Value of Each Outcome

The final phase of the decision analysis process is to assess the desirability of the various outcomes. The joint probabilities are calculated by multiplying all of the probabilities along a particular branch. The joint probabilities give the probability of occurrence for each potential outcome or end point on the tree.

Next, a numerical value, known as *utility*, is assigned to the various outcomes. Utility represents a preference for one outcome over others. In health care, some outcomes are clearly desirable (for example, increased quality delivered at a lower price). In the MRI example, the utility is based on the expected profitability or expected monetary value (EV) of each outcome. Clearly, the desired outcome in this example is a market share increase of 20 percent, resulting in an incremental profit of $2 million.

Utility is often not black or white. Not all outcomes can be based on financial performance or mathematical assignment. For example, for certain patients with cancer of the larynx, survival is better for those who have radical surgery than for those treated with radiotherapy. However, radical surgery limits the ability to speak in the short run. Therefore, there is a trade-off between survival, which is maximized by surgery, and the ability to communicate, which is more likely retained with radiotherapy (Lilford, Parker, Braunholtz, and Chard, 1998).

Accounting for Uncertainty:
Ongoing Monitoring and Contingency Planning

As discussed throughout this book, even those who recognize uncertainty tend to underestimate its ongoing impact. Most organizations compete in uncertain environments by using strategies that, though justified when launched, lose their validity as business conditions change (Kaplan and Norton, 1996b). Decision trees amount to a map illustrating the evolution of possible actions, outcomes, probabilities, and expected impacts. This road map allows decision makers to monitor the progress of the situation, and to make revisions as necessary in response to "wrong turns." Furthermore, the expected value calculation is useful in determining how much the decision maker should be willing to invest to increase the odds of a desired outcome.

In an attempt to learn from experience, organizations and individuals tend to focus on the consequences of decisions made in the past. However, any of a number of chance, uncontrollable factors can lead to the final outcome. Although the past is sometimes a good predictor of the future, decision makers may rely too heavily on past experiences. It is worthwhile to consider George Santayana's words ("Those who do not remember the past are condemned to relive it"), but it is true also that in an attempt to avoid making the same mistake twice we often avoid a previously chosen course of action, even though it would be the right decision the second time (Dawes, 1988).

In addition to constant monitoring of the environment, and making subsequent adjustments, organizations must have a backup or contingency plan in place. Although essential in an uncertain environment, contingency planning is rarely undertaken by health care organizations. Organizations need to prepare for the possibility that expected outcomes may not materialize, on account of unforeseen or unexpected events.

Benefits and Drawbacks of Decision Analysis

Decision analysis allows an organization to understand the consequences of a decision and incorporate this knowledge into the decision-making process. It can help in forecasting the likely impact of potential decisions in an environment where discrete alternatives exist. Decision analysis also:

- Clarifies potential combinations of alternatives

- Clearly communicates options available from various decisions

- Allows an organization to anticipate future decisions and use this knowledge to make better decisions early in the process

- Allows an organization to clearly identify controllable and noncontrollable elements and see at what points it does or does not have control

- Promotes understanding of how change may occur

- Allows calculation of the expected value of a decision

Decision analysis is appropriate whenever discrete alternatives exist, probabilities can be reasonably assessed, and a potential outcome can have a significant impact on the organization. Like all tools, decision analysis does not work in all situations. Decision trees were not designed to model uncertainty with a wide range of futures. The role of judgment and intuition cannot be ignored in the decision analysis framework. Using decision analysis tools to automate the decision process, impose solutions, or predefine objectives without input from leaders results in misguided decisions.

Decision analysis is often viewed as unemotional and obsessive because it is a quantitative approach to decision making. Indeed, decision analysis can be extended too far where using numbers is inappropriate. For example, how can a measure be placed on quality of life? Despite its limitations, when used as a complementary tool in the planning process decision analysis has been shown to be effective in clarifying options and structuring uncertainties to improve decision making.

Game Theory

Scenario planning helps to synthesize a broad range of alternatives, and decision analysis clarifies the likely outcomes of a few discrete alternatives. **Game theory** is a planning tool that helps managers understand their strategic options in the context of other related parties—specifically, customers, competitors, strategic partners, and suppliers. This tool is particularly useful in helping to understand and reduce uncertainty about how the actions and reactions of other entities affect the organization.

History and Applications of Game Theory

Game theory is the branch of social science that studies strategic thinking and decision making as an interactive process among interrelated parties. John von Neumann developed the foundations of game theory in the late 1920s. Game theory as a formal science was pioneered in the 1940s and further evolved through mathematics. It gained popularity after three scholars of game theory were awarded the Nobel Prize in 1994.

Although game theory was originally applied to situations of military conflict, it can provide insight into a wide range of situations, from chess to child rearing, and has recently been applied successfully to business strategy. Here is a health care case that illustrates several key principles of game theory.

Hospital A, located in a rural area, is seeking to join a large system. Hospital A has a historical "working relationship" with Hospital B. A views B as the logical partner and asks it to develop a merger proposal. The key question for Hospital A is, "How can we leverage our negotiating position?" Its answer is to bring in another player.

A asks Hospital C, a for-profit hospital and major competitor of B's, to develop a merger proposal. As a result, A's improved negotiating position allows it to secure a "fair" partnership with B.

In this example, Hospital A applies two principles of game theory that are be discussed further in this chapter: allocentrism (putting yourself in others' shoes), and changing the game by adding players.

Defining the Game

Before decision makers can apply game theory in strategic decision making, they must understand the basic framework. A "game" is any situation of strategic interdependence. The five primary elements in any game can be summarized by the acronym PARTS (players, added values, rules, tactics, and scope; Brandenburger and Nalebuff, 1995):

- Players: customers, suppliers, competitors, and complementors. (These players are described further in the next section, on the value net.)

- Added value: what each player brings to the game; it is the primary source of power for each player. Each player's added value is equal to the size of the whole pie when the player is in the game minus the size of the pie when the player is out of the game.

- Rules: rules give structure to the game. Rules vary by industry and market and may change at any time.

- Tactics: moves used to shape how a player perceives the game.

- Scope: the boundaries of the game. Like rules, scope is not constant and is subject to continuous revision.

Understanding the Value Net

In a game, players must create or add value before they can capture it. Value creation is often best achieved through the cooperation of multiple parties. The term *value net* is used to describe the various players (the P in PARTS) in the game and their interdependency (Brandenburger and Nalebuff, 1995). Competitors, complementors, customers, and suppliers are all included in an organization's value net. If your product is more valued when another player's product is involved, that player is a complementor. For example, if a prestigious hospital recruits the city's premier cardiovascular physician group, the two players are complementors. Conversely, if your product or service is valued less when another player's product is involved, that player is a competitor. If the prestigious hospital must share the cardiovascular group with another hospital that recently initiated open-heart surgery, the two hospitals are competitors. It can be extremely valuable to bring new players into the value net because each player adds value to the game, increasing the size of the whole pie. In the world of technology, Microsoft and Intel each are much better off because they both exist in one another's value net.

There are both competition and cooperation within a value net. It is possible for players to simultaneously occupy more than one role. For the earlier example, the cardiovascular physician group can simultaneously be a competitor and a complementor. American Airlines and Delta Airlines typically compete against each other for airline passengers, but they also complement each other. Since both airlines are supplied airplanes by Boeing, it is much cheaper for Boeing to design planes for the two airlines simultaneously. If Boeing can split the development costs between the two airlines, it is a win-win situation for American and Delta (Brandenburger and Nalebuff, 1995).

As shown in Figure 5.3, hospitals, physicians, and payers play multiple roles in a hospital's value net. The strong economic power of physicians is apparent from their appearing in all four areas of the health care value net. As a customer, a complementor, and a competitor in a hospital's value net, payers also have significant influence.

Useful Lessons from Game Theory

Game theory teaches us four basic lessons that help us reduce uncertainty and understand how other entities' decisions might affect our organization.

Lesson One: To Every Action There Is a Reaction

One of the fundamental concepts of game theory is that no one operates in a vacuum. Any strategy or tactic that affects another player is likely to prompt a reaction. For example, when Columbia Healthcare pursued its aggressive "national dominance" strategy in the mid-1990s, many regional community hospitals banded together in response and formed unexpectedly strong coalitions. In 1992, there were nine independent hospitals operating in Charleston, South Carolina. Largely due to the threat Columbia posed locally, by year's end 1999 only one of these hospitals remained independent (Kichheimer, 1999). Other players, such as suppliers and customers, can react too. The Health Care Financing Administration (HCFA) decision to limit increases for Medicare HMO payments at a time of rising pharmacy and provider costs led to a steady stream of HMOs pulling out of unprofitable markets in 1998 and 1999. In essence, HCFA sabotaged its own strategy of shifting Medicare enrollees into managed care plans to control costs.

Lesson Two: Added Value

A player can't take more away from the game than it brings. The concept of added value is critical because it determines the amount

Figure 5.3. Players in the Health Care Value Net.

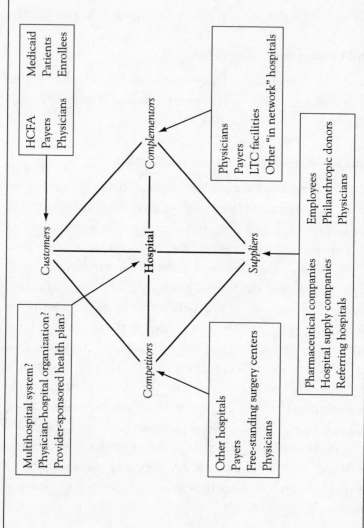

Source: Adapted and reprinted by permission of *Harvard Business Review*, exhibit "Who Are the Players in Your Company's Value Net?" from "The Right Game: Use Game Theory to Shape Strategy" by A. M. Brandenburger and B. J. Nalebuff, July–Aug. 1995, p. 60. Copyright ©1995 by the President and Fellows of Harvard College; all rights reserved.

of power each player has in interactions and defines the value that the player can extract from the interaction. In the affiliation example at the beginning of this section, Hospital A increases its added value in the negotiations by changing the scope of the game from a two-party negotiation to a three-party one. By inviting Hospital B's competitor into the game, A increases its own added value.

Lesson Three: Allocentrism

"When I am getting ready to reason with a man," Abraham Lincoln advised us, "I spend one-third of my time thinking about what I am going to say and two-thirds thinking about what he is going to say."

The primary insight of game theory is the importance of focusing on others, which is known as allocentrism. A thief who is debating whether to rob banks (because that's where the money is) or convenience stores must know that the police are asking themselves "What type of establishment would I target if I were a thief?" and should act accordingly (Davis, 1983). An egocentric view, that is, one from the thief's point of view, says to rob the bank, as the payoff is higher. An allocentric view considers the thoughts of the police and realizes that chances of getting caught at the bank are much greater. Although we cannot tell with certainty which is a better option for the thief, his or her chances of being caught are far less in deciding to target convenience stores.

In the health care industry, hospital executives must consider the potential reactions of managed care companies before launching provider-based managed care products. Similarly, regional referral hospitals need to consider how outlying referring hospitals react to development of ambulatory satellite centers in their backyard.

Role playing can be an effective exercise in improving allocentric thinking. To facilitate a role-playing exercise, assign people to play such roles as specific competitors, customers, and suppliers; articulate the perceptions, needs, expectations, and biases of each. Then, play through the situation, using the tools of negotiation, or marketing strategy, with each player making decisions that are in its own best interest.

Lesson Four: Zero-Sum Games Versus "Co-Opetition"

In "zero-sum games," such as football and poker, one player's gain is another player's loss and the players have no common interests. On the other hand, in a fully cooperative game, the players have nothing but common interests. An example of full cooperation is two sailboats maneuvering to avoid a collision (Davis, 1983). Most situations fall somewhere in between and include both cooperation and competition. This situation has been termed "co-opetition." In a co-opetitive environment, one player may not have to lose in order for another to win. Ray Noorda, founder of Novell, who coined the term *co-opetition,* is said to have declared that "business is cooperation when it comes to creating a pie and competition when it comes to dividing it up. You have to compete and cooperate at the same time."

Health care is flush with examples of co-opetition, in part because of the high interdependency among players. Hospitals and health systems, payers, and physicians are all interdependent. One of the big health care stories of the 1990s was the proliferation of alliances among "competitor" hospitals to create a bigger pie by negotiating higher payment rates from managed care companies. In Atlanta, managed care organizations began collaborating with each other in developing common practice guidelines. Although "the intense competition among plans almost thwarted plans for collaboration," managed care companies realized "if all plans are promoting the same preventive health programs, they won't fear losing on their investment if their members disenroll" ("Atlanta MCOs Collaborating . . . ," 1999, p. 3).

Game Theory Strategy

Game theory gives us several useful rules to reduce some of the uncertainty surrounding strategy formulation.

Rule One: Look Forward and Reason Backward

Game theory is a tool for making decisions, but before you decide how to get what you want you must first decide specifically what it is that you want. Once this is determined, look to the endgame and reason backward from the desired outcome.

Rule Two: If You Have a Dominant Strategy, Use It

A dominant strategy makes a player better off than he or she would be with any other strategy, no matter what strategy the opponent uses.

A baseball example illustrates this. You are the manager of a baseball team, and your team is up to bat. It's the bottom of the ninth inning. The bases are loaded. There are two outs, and the count stands at three balls and two strikes. What do you signal the base runners to do? Under any potential outcome, the best decision is to steal home (Dixit and Nalebuff, 1991).

If opening a satellite ambulatory surgery center is more profitable than adding operating rooms to the hospital campus regardless of how the competition reacts, the organization should pursue this dominant strategy.

Rule Three: Eliminate Dominated Strategies from Consideration

A dominated strategy is one that is uniformly worse than another potential strategy, regardless of the actions of competitors. Using the ambulatory surgery center example, adding operating rooms on the hospital campus is the dominated strategy, since the outcome is inferior regardless of what the competition does. Once a strategy has been identified as a dominant or dominated strategy, it's easy to decide whether to pursue it. The trick is to identify early which strategies are dominant and which are dominated.

Rule Four: Look for Equilibrium

Remembering that one organization need not fail for another to succeed, strive for equilibrium, which creates a sustainable situation. Seek the equilibrium that results in greatest benefit to each party.

Consider this health care adaptation of the classic Prisoner's Dilemma. A hospital is considering developing a provider sponsored organization (PSO). The hospital realizes that this is a risky move, but it is seriously considering this option because the dominant HMO in the market is offering very unattractive payment rates. The hospital is in the process of negotiating with the HMO to obtain more favorable rates, but the outcome of the talks is uncertain. Assume that the hospital's and HMO's profits are based on the outcome of the hospital's PSO development and the HMO's payment decisions. This situation is illustrated in Figure 5.4.

From an independent viewpoint and ignoring the decision of the other player, the hospital's best option is to develop the PSO, while the HMO's most attractive choice is to maintain current payment rates. Assuming that the players are not working together cooperatively, both the hospital and the HMO should go with their dominant strategies. This results in a profit of $10 million for each party. However, if the hospital and HMO employ their dominant strategies, the two players would be better off looking for the equilibrium. The resulting payoff at the equilibrium is $12 million in profit for each.

Figure 5.4. Analysis of PSO Development Options.

		HMO's Choices			
		Raise payment rates		Do not raise payment rates	
		Hospital	*HMO*	*Hospital*	*HMO*
Hospital's Choices	Develop PSO	$16 million	$4 million	$10 million	$10 million
	Do not develop PSO	$12 million	$12 million	$8 million	$16 million

Rule Five: Change the Game

Players can change the game by altering any of its components. Examples include bringing in new players (here, cardiologists inviting MedCath into the market, changing the rules by influencing health care legislation, or broadening scope by adding a financing component to a delivery system). Deciding whether the organization should change the game, and if so, how, are discussed fully in Chapter Six.

Game Theory as a Planning Tool

Applying game theory is particularly relevant in an era of uncertainty because it permits organizations to make strategic decisions within an allocentric framework. It identifies the players, specifies the options available to each player, establishes payoffs for every combination of options, and facilitates rational decision making by defining sequences of decisions. It offers predictive power and allows insight into situations of competition and bargaining.

Game theory is unique and effective because it recognizes explicitly that in any game there are others present who are making decisions. Their decisions are based on what they believe results in their success. Anticipating their response can give a health care organization a competitive advantage in strategy formulation. Internally, it can be used to explain to others why certain decisions are made. In a broad sense, game theory lets an organization see what is happening and what actions can be taken in response.

Game theory is used most appropriately when two or more organizations' success is interdependent. The benefits of game theory are best realized when competitors' alternatives are discrete. Game theory may be difficult to apply if the issue at hand involves many competitors or competitors have a wide range of options.

Conclusion

The tools discussed in this chapter—scenario planning, decision analysis, and game theory—are the means to an end, not an end unto themselves. They are part of the larger planning process included in phase two of the strategy cycle (identifying the nature and extent of residual uncertainties). These tools draw on the information gathered through developing the environmental assessment (Chapter Three) and the planning assumptions (Chapter Four). The main purpose of these new planning tools is to help synthesize and weigh complex and uncertain environmental factors so that decision makers may formulate the organization's strategic intent (the subject of Chapter Six).

As discussed throughout this chapter, the three new planning tools are appropriate for certain circumstances and have their own benefits and drawbacks. Table 5.1 summarizes these differences.

Lessons Learned
• •

✓ A new set of planning tools, widely used in the corporate world, is available to help health care leaders understand and reduce the increasing uncertainty of environmental factors.

✓ Scenario planning helps to organize and reduce uncertainty by synthesizing large amounts of data into a limited number of possible stories that are easy to understand.

✓ Decision analysis helps to organize and reduce uncertainty by clearly identifying controllable and noncontrollable elements and mapping expected outcomes of decision alternatives.

✓ Game theory helps to reduce the uncertainty related to the actions of external parties by permitting a framework for understanding interdependencies among players.

Table 5.1. Comparison of Planning Tools to Address Uncertainty.

Tool	When to Use It	Benefits	Drawbacks
Scenario planning	When levels of uncertainty are high for several critically important variables When key uncertainties are not easily segregated into discrete alternatives	Synthesizes large amounts of information into limited number of future states Challenges conventional wisdom and broadens leaders' perspectives	Easy to misuse as a predictive tool Subjective in nature, built on participant biases
Decision analysis	When discrete alternatives exist and probabilities can be reasonably assessed When the organization prefers a quantitative approach to decision making	Maps future consequences of decisions Quantifies the impact of decisions by factoring in controllable and uncontrollable circumstances	Not applicable for uncertainties containing a wide range of alternatives Rigid structure gives little consideration to judgment and intuition
Game theory	When the decision is heavily influenced by potential actions of other parties	Creates a framework for managing uncertainty related to the actions of other organizations	Not appropriate if issue involves many players with wide range of options

6

Defining Strategic Intent

Deborah S. Kolb and Kathleen Rausch Henchey

W hy spend time developing a vision for the future if the present is so uncertain? Faced with the same set of market circumstances, why do two competing organizations make very different choices? This chapter explains the critical strategic planning component, "strategic intent," which describes the organization's identity and future vision. We explore the key components of strategic intent as well as the forms it can take, using health care and other industry examples as illustrations. The chapter concludes with advice on a process and tools to assist the organization in establishing its strategic intent.

What Is Strategic Intent?

"Know thyself." In times of great change and uncertainty, both individuals and organizations are well advised to pause and reflect on what truly matters to them. In the first two phases of the strategy cycle (Figure 2.3), the organization focuses on understanding external market forces and its starting position. Now, in phase three, attention is turned inward as an organization examines its core being—what it is, where it wants to go, and how it will get there. This process is called "defining strategic intent."

Faced with the same set of market conditions, organizations will head in varying directions. Strategic intent is what differentiates organizations from one another and causes them to choose alternative paths. Strategic intent encompasses an organization's corporate identity, envisioned future direction, and tolerance for risk. It comprises three distinct but interrelated components: core ideology, vision, and market stance (Table 6.1).

Before it can develop strategies for the future, an organization must first know why it exists. Every firm has a **core ideology,** a cultural identity that transcends the services it offers and the people who work for it (Collins and Porras, 1996). This core ideology fundamentally shapes where the organization chooses to go and how it chooses to get there. An organization's core ideology is expressed formally in its core purpose and its values.

Core purpose is an organization's reason for being. At most health care organizations, this core purpose is captured in the **mission** statement. For example, the mission statement of an integrated delivery system might be "To improve the health of the people of our community." A Catholic health care system's mission statement might read "Our mission is to work together and with others to continue the health ministry of the Church, promoting the well-being

Table 6.1. The Three Components of Strategic Intent.

Question	Answer	Characteristics
Who are we?	Core ideology	Core purpose and mission Core values
Where do we want to go?	Vision	Statement that is succinct, compelling, and easy to communicate Differentiates the organization from the competition
How will we get there?	Market stance	Degree of market uncertainty Risk preference Corporate culture Current strategic position Financial capacity

of the people in the communities we serve." A children's hospital's mission statement might be "To enhance the lives of children through excellence in patient care, research, and education."

Core values are those intrinsic beliefs that the organization cherishes above all others. These values are inherent in the organization; they characterize the best efforts of the organization throughout changing market conditions. For example, the core values of Catholic Health East are reverence for each person, community, justice, commitment to those who are poor, stewardship, courage, and integrity (Catholic Health East, 1999). Advocate Health Care in Chicago values equality, compassion, excellence, partnership, and stewardship (Advocate Health Care, 1998). An organization's core values may be expressed in a values statement, but just as often they are acted upon rather than explicitly stated.

A solid understanding of core ideology enables the organization to determine its **vision,** the second component of strategic intent. A vision statement describes where the organization wants to go. To be effective, a vision statement should be succinct, compelling, and easy to communicate. It should also differentiate the company from its competitors. One vision statement that imparts such a clear focus is from Michael Farrell, Senior Vice President of Administrative Services at Children's Healthcare of Atlanta: "Be the model for addressing children's health needs by defining, then providing or advocating for: accessible, innovative and excellent patient care; integrated teaching and research; and partnership in wellness and prevention programs."

Some organizations never articulate a clear vision. Other organizations make the mistake of putting too many ideas into a vision statement, leaving those who are charged with implementing it bewildered about where to start. John P. Kotter, who has assisted many corporate change efforts, cites lack of a clear vision as one of the main reasons companies fail to implement change (1995).

The third component of strategic intent is the organization's **market stance,** or how it goes about realizing its vision. An organization's market stance depends on a combination of factors: the degree of uncertainty characterizing the market in which it operates (as discerned in phase two of the strategic planning process); the nature and level of risk it is willing to assume; its corporate culture; and its current strategic position and capabilities, including financial capacity.

Basic Forms of Strategic Intent

An organization's primary strategic intent can be conceptualized as taking one of three basic forms: "market enactor," "market adapter," or "market survivor" (adapted from Courtney, Kirkland, and Viguerie, 1997). These three approaches vary according to the organization's core ideology, its vision, and its market stance. Most organizations have one dominant form of strategic intent, although they incorporate selected strategies across the three basic forms of intent in their plan (Table 6.2).

Descriptions of the three basic forms of intent are provided below.

The Market Enactor

The **market enactor** approaches uncertainty by trying to change the world to its strategic advantage. Enactors seek to change the nature of competition and to force competitors to react to their moves. To use a nautical metaphor, a market enactor is a powerful steamship that generates a great wake. However, it cannot easily change direction once it has set its course.

The core ideology of a market enactor embraces action and leadership. Successful market enactors have a proactive orientation, relishing their role in shaping the market's direction as well as anticipating market changes. A successful market enactor has an entrepreneurial organizational culture and leaders who emphasize and reward innovation and prudent risk taking (Kolb, 1996). Often, a market enactor has a culture dominated by a visionary leader who is authoritarian in setting direction. A market enactor's leadership

Table 6.2. Basic Forms of Strategic Intent.

Form	Characteristics	Accompanied by	Level of Risk
Market enactor	Lead industry structure, standards, change	"Big bet" moves Risk-taking leaders Financial strength "Staying the course"	High
Market adapter	Prevail with agility in recognizing and capitalizing on all opportunities	Flexibility and willingness to change course (identify exit strategies up front) Hedge bets Attention to new technologies	Medium
Market survivor	Stay in the game, but avoid premature commitments	"No regrets" moves Positioning as desirable partner Incremental moves focused on infrastructure and customers	Low

is committed to stay the course in the face of adversity but willing to occasionally make radical changes if market indicators reveal the need for reassessment. Market enactors are willing to move forward without full consensus. They also expect and accept some failures along the way.

In its vision, the market enactor seeks not only to establish a leading market position but to change how the game is played—or even to create new game rules. For example, a market-enacting health care system may develop a system ready for capitation long before the market demands it, accelerating the market's move to managed care. Expressing one overarching organizational goal can catalyze the market-enacting organization. Tracy Goss and colleagues emphasize the value of a "declaration" statement, clearly describing where the company wants to go. "When a declaration is well stated, it is always visually imaginable (NASA's 'putting a man on the moon') or exceptionally simple (British Airways' 'becoming the world's favourite airline')" (Goss, Pascale, and Athos, 1998, p. 97).

The market enactor's high tolerance for risk is evident in its market stance. The enactor often chooses risky, big-bet approaches that can create big payoffs but that also carry real downside risk. Although a market enactor may be aware of uncertainty in the environment, it chooses its course based on preferences and vision. This approach requires a strong financial position, which allows the organization to commit the resources necessary to initiate and sustain its strategies. A risk-averse organization cannot be a successful market enactor. Given their fiduciary responsibilities to the community, most not-for-profit organizations tend to be relatively risk-averse; therefore, there are few market enactors among health care systems.

In any industry, the fact is that true market enactors are rare. It takes a considerable amount of skill, resources, foresight, and probably luck to redirect the course of a market. As described in Chapter Two, FedEx is a classic example of a successful market enactor. Its introduction of overnight delivery service fundamentally shifted consumers' expectations about mail service. Many of today's Internet companies—such as eBay, the online auction house, and drugstore.com, the online pharmacy—are aspiring market enactors. In the health care industry, Humana's decision to enter the insurance business, and then later to divest its core hospital business, is characteristic of a market enactor. Sentara Healthcare has successfully enacted its market in southeastern Virginia and northeastern North Carolina by developing a full continuum of branded health care services linked with HMOs and physician foundations.

Of course, not all market enactors are successful. The collapse of the Allegheny Health Education Research Foundation (AHERF) in Pennsylvania presents a sobering reminder that **big bets** are not for the faint of heart. On the premise that bigger is better, AHERF rapidly acquired hospitals and physician practices in a big-bet strategy founded on capitation and the PCP gatekeeper model. AHERF demonstrated myriad other strategic and operational missteps, but its declaration of bankruptcy in July 1998 stunned health care systems across the country, many of which had developed the same set of planning assumptions and were implementing similar, though smaller-scale, strategies.

The experience of the Laura Ashley company demonstrates how market enactors that fail to monitor changing markets can find themselves moving full steam in the wrong direction (Sull, 1999). Laura Ashley exemplifies the visionary founder characteristic of many market enactors. She had a unique vision and set of values that evoked nostalgia and romance. She based her production in Britain and bestowed generous wages and benefits. Women flocked to her fashions, and the company expanded rapidly throughout the 1970s. By the early 1980s, however, the fashion industry had changed. More women were entering the workforce and choosing professional, tailored clothing. Most apparel manufacturers moved their factories offshore to lower production costs. Instead, the company brought in a series of CEOs, all of whom initiated small, incremental changes such as programs to increase sales and cut costs. None of these seven CEOs went far enough in recasting the fundamental vision and strategy of the company. It was time to rethink the founder's vision.

The Market Adapter

A **market adapter** favors strategies tailored to a best guess about the direction of the market, while keeping options open. To continue the nautical metaphor, the market adapter is a sleek sailing ship, fast and agile, adapting quickly to changes in the weather. Unlike the market enactor, it generates little wake for its competitors.

Flexibility is the hallmark of the market adapter. These organizations exhibit ongoing attentiveness to market changes and new technologies, coupled with willingness and ability to change course quickly. The culture of the market adapter is one of acceptance of, and willingness to learn from, mistakes. Its decision-making processes are systematic and analytically based. Critically important, the market adapter is willing to exit a market or service if necessary.

The market adapter's management model is one of delegation and empowerment to act on market opportunities, typically using ad hoc work teams and partnerships with other organizations. The market adapting organization values high-performing work teams that have a high degree of "emotional intelligence" (Goleman, 1997). When successful, these work teams allow the talents of individual members to flourish.

Like the market enactor, the market adapter has a clear vision of where it wants to go. The difference lies in their market stances. The primary strategy of the market adapter is to prevail with agility until there is more certainty about the direction of the market. Unlike a market enactor, which changes some of the rules of the game or even creates smaller new games, market adapters are likely to hedge their bets by adopting less risky strategies that can be modified as the market or the rules of the game change. For example, where a market enactor might choose to own an insurance company in order to exert control, a market adapter might limit its capital exposure through a joint venture, identifying exit strategies up front.

Although a market adapter does not require the financial resources of a market enactor, it still needs sufficient financial capacity to redirect expenditures as necessary to respond to market opportunities. Typically, the organization has a large cash cushion but chooses not to risk a major portion of its reserves if there is a high degree of uncertainty.

Many large, successful companies are market adapters. They watch new trends and wait to see if they take hold before investing resources. Market adapters leverage other organizations' achievements. The fast-food industry illustrates the difference between the market enactor and the market adapter. McDonald's was a market enactor, creating a new demand for meals that were fast and of consistent quality. By the 1990s, however, consumers wanted different, healthier fast-food options. Burger King and Taco Bell, both market adapters, recognized this market shift and offered new menu options, eroding McDonald's market position. In the personal computer (PC) industry, market enactor Dell Computer has outdistanced rivals IBM and Compaq by selling PCs directly to customers, first by mail order and then over the Internet. Gateway and other adapters followed in Dell's wake (Sull, 1999).

Often, not-for-profit health care organizations are market adapters. They may not be the first to have a primary care physician network or managed care product, but they develop them if they see that others have been successful. Health care market adapters include the integrated delivery systems that are entering into partnerships with online medical advice websites, such as AmericasDoctor.com.

The Market Survivor

A third form of strategic intent is to wait until the environment becomes more certain. This **market-survivor** approach may become the de facto strategy: even if an organization wants to adopt an assertive market posture, it may wind up here if it cannot achieve agreement about market direction or is saddled with a corporate culture that is paralyzed in the face of an uncertain future. As with market adapters, market survivors may have a clear vision but lack certainty about market stance. If the market enactors and adapters are, nautically speaking, already at sea, then market survivors are best described as back at the dock with the boat ready to go, waiting for weather conditions to change.

To survive, an organization must have a winning operational focus and sufficient financial resources to allow it to stay in the game. At the same time, it must be attentive to changes in the market that signal the need to reset strategy, and be willing to change course accordingly.

The market survivor usually has a track record of success, the need to feel in control of its strategies, and low tolerance for risk.

Playing by the current set of game rules, it tries to outperform the competition. This type of organization typically invests in **"no-regrets moves,"** such as improving infrastructure and customer focus, reducing costs, and improving quality. These incremental, operational moves are important to the ongoing success of any organization, but they are not substitutes for strategy, which involves making choices about where and how to compete. A common market stance of the market survivor is to shore up the organization's weaknesses to position it as a desirable partner.

Many hospitals and health care systems are in this category. The rapid pace of change and uncertainty about the market have immobilized them, rendering them unable to set a definitive strategic course. Ironically, by waiting, some organizations have avoided the damaging storms that rocked so many health care systems that heeded siren calls such as physician practice acquisition or HMO development.

To understand the differences among these three forms of strategic intent, imagine three hospitals in a market with these characteristics: increasing managed care penetration; physician group formation; and the potential entry of a for-profit, niche competitor. A market enactor might seek to acquire one of the managed care plans to have more control over the managed care market and to fortify its position relative to the niche competitor. A market adapter might develop innovative partnership models with key physician groups, regularly assessing the models' effectiveness for all parties. A market survivor might focus on improving its patient satisfaction scores and reducing its costs until it sees how the market sorts out.

Issues in Defining Strategic Intent

Each organization has a dominant form of strategic intent, but divisions or service lines within the organization may have differing strategic intent. For example, an organization might react to overall market uncertainty by taking a wait-and-see approach at a system level but choose to enact the market in a strong service line in which it feels there is more certainty. Another organization may be a skilled market adapter in most services but adopt a market survivor approach in a particular area of great residual uncertainty, such as home health services or physician practice acquisition.

Given today's dynamic, uncertain health care market, an organization should expect to refine its strategic intent at least every three years—more frequently, if there are compelling market events. Market enactors that do not heed trigger points may find themselves pursuing a precarious direction. Market survivors need to be watchful of their opportunities to get into the game.

It is challenging to define strategic intent for complex health care organizations with many lines of business and multiple consumers. For an integrated delivery system with six acute care hospitals, a psychiatric hospital, three skilled nursing facilities, a home health agency, and an HMO, it can be hard to identify what truly unifies it. Size and scale can help an organization weather market storms, but as American industry learned in the 1980s, unless driven by unity of purpose an unfocused conglomerate may be better off dismantled (Governance Institute, 1996). As described in Chapter Five, game theory is a useful tool for thinking about strategic intent in complex organizations. Members of the planning committee of an integrated delivery system should ask themselves, "What is the added value that we bring to the table, given all the possible players competing in our marketplace?"

Not-for-profit health care organizations face special challenges in defining strategic intent. Whereas a for-profit company seeks to leverage its position to benefit the shareholders, the typical mission of the not-for-profit organization makes it responsible and accountable to the community as a whole. The traditional role that the not-for-profit hospital has played in serving a geographically defined community makes it unlikely that it will adopt "bet the farm" strategies that endanger its long-term ability to continue to serve the community.

Because it frequently results in awareness of the need for change, the process of determining strategic intent is seldom a comfortable one. Change is alarming for everyone involved: trustees, management, physicians, and employees. Compounding the problem, companies are full of "change survivors," who have seen many change efforts and are skeptical of new ones (Duck, 1998). As we shall see in Chapter Nine, the organization's leaders must be prepared to establish the need to change and engender enthusiasm for a shared vision. Leaders need to set the example by living the vision: people believe it if they see it in action, not just on paper. Consider, for example, a hospital that commits itself to the highest quality in customer service. What message is the CEO sending if his or her office is in a remote part of the hospital, or even off-site? Does he or she regularly walk the halls and greet employees by name? Contrast this with another CEO who sets the example for customer service by having a central, accessible office; takes the time to speak with employees and patients; and guides lost visitors to their destinations. The adage holds: actions speak louder than words.

Regardless of an organization's particular strategic intent, several critical success factors are shared. The first is commitment to mission, which is understood throughout the organization and forms the foundation against which all decisions are measured. The second is a vision that differentiates this organization from its competitors. The third is clear, widely shared understanding of the organization's strategic intent. Everyone in the organization should be able to describe the company's mission, vision, and values. Fourth, there needs to be broad support for the organization's strategic intent among employees, trustees, physicians, and community leaders. The fifth success factor is ongoing use of no-regrets moves, such as continuous improvements in cost and quality. Although these are not substitutes for strategy, all organizations must engage in these activities to stay in the game. Last but not least, financial capacity is a key critical success factor to realizing strategic intent.

As discussed in Chapter Eight, organizations must candidly assess their ability to fund new ventures and sustain operations. Strategic intent and **financial capability** are interdependent; strategic intent drives allocation of scarce resources, but financial resources can ultimately constrain or enable strategic intent.

The Process of Defining Strategic Intent

The process of defining strategic intent involves articulating core ideology, that is, the core purpose and core values, the vision, and the market stance. To define its strategic intent, an organization must start with the core purpose. Careful reading of the mission statement is a good place to start; this statement describes an organization's reason for being. Chances are the mission statement will remain intact; nevertheless, it is important to revisit it to ensure that the mission describes the organization's core purpose.

Identifying the fundamental tenets that guide an organization is also critical in defining strategic intent, because an organization cannot enact a vision and market stance that are at odds with its internal corporate culture. An organization's core values may not be as accessible or explicitly defined as its core purpose. These five to six core values are ones that the organization cherishes above all others and that have endured the test of time. To identify what really matters to an organization, the planning committee should draft a preliminary list of values, avoiding buzzwords such as *quality* and *excellence* and instead using expressions that are clear and compelling. For example, one of Nordstrom's core values is "service to the customer above all else." Other companies have more unusual tenets, such as Walt Disney's "no cynicism," or Sony's "elevation of the Japanese culture and national status." For each entry on the list, the committee needs to ask, "If circumstances changed and penalized us for holding this core value, would we keep it?" If the answer is no, then this is not a core value (Collins and Porras, 1996).

The next step in defining strategic intent is to develop a vision for the organization. A vision statement is one of imagination and foresight that describes a desired future: "Where do we want to be in three to five years?" Many health care organizations have created vision statements at some point. If one exists, the planning committee should reexamine the organization's vision statement to evaluate its continued relevance. If well-crafted, a vision should stretch the goals of the organization and offer a vivid picture of where it is headed. Avoid the temptation to put too many ideas into a vision statement. Instead, focus on a clear picture of where you want to take your organization. A weak vision statement is one whose text fills an entire page. A good vision statement energizes the organization: "Our vision is to be internationally recognized as a leader in innovative cancer research."

The last step in developing strategic intent is to consider the organization's preferred market stance. Market enactors are aggressive risk takers. With strong, often autocratic leadership and significant financial capability, they are willing to assume greater risks in return for greater payoffs as they strive to change the market. Market adapters assume less risk but make certain they are able to respond quickly to market opportunities by decentralizing leadership and maintaining financial reserves for new strategic initiatives. Market survivors are the type least comfortable with risk. Often burdened by limited financial capability, their leaders concentrate on making operational improvements and shoring up their resources.

The process of defining strategic intent takes time. When spread over a number of meetings, it may take several months to define core ideology, vision, and market stance. An all-day retreat is one way to speed up and consolidate the process. Whichever approach is used, it is important to structure the process carefully, encourage participation, and make progress during each session.

Once the planning committee has defined strategic intent, its members will want to review the recommendations with key stakeholders throughout the organization, including trustees, physicians, community leaders, and employees. The greater the clarity about strategic intent, the easier this communication process is.

Facilitating Discussions of Market Stance

In our experience, a facilitation tool known as creating a **new path** is a particularly effective and engaging tool that can help an organization define its market stance (McWhinney and others, 1993).

The "game board" is a visual representation of the various dimensions of the organization's characteristics, services, and relationships. For each dimension, alternative strategies can be pursued. Current market stance is plotted alongside preferred market stance, to highlight where the organization is changing course. This tool is also helpful for subsequently setting measures of success in phase four of the strategy cycle (described in Chapter Seven).

Creating a New Path in a Health Care System

We now present a simplified illustration of a seven-step process to create a new path for a health care system. Our example focuses on five dimensions that are critical for the system's success:

1. Horizontal integration

2. Primary care physician integration

3. Managed care partners

4. Managed care pricing

5. Geographic focus

Your organization is likely to have a different set of issues or concerns. Most organizations examine six to ten dimensions to create a complete picture of their preferred intent and stance.

Step One: Create the Game Board

As a group, list the key dimensions of market stance for your organization across the top of the page. These dimensions should be aspects of the organization that emerge as critical issues from the confidential interviews, in the environmental assessment, during development of the planning assumptions, or in considering the major uncertainties the organization faces. For each dimension, list the alternative approaches available to you in the appropriate column. Many of these alternatives are ones you have identified during phase two of the strategy cycle. Each alternative should represent a distinct way of addressing the dimension. For example, in Figure 6.1, horizontal integration includes a range of options, from a fully merged multihospital health system to an informal network of relationships.

Step Two: Describe the Current Approach and the Preferred Alternative

For every dimension, each individual selects the alternative that best matches what the organization is currently doing. Then the individual selects the alternative he or she believes to be the preferred one. Note that the current choice and the preferred approach can be the same for any dimension. Forcing a selection among alternatives is a valuable exercise. As noted by Michael Porter, "Strategy is making trade-offs in competing. The essence of strategy is choosing what not to do. Without trade-offs, there would be no need for choice and thus no need for strategy" (Porter, 1996, p. 70).

Step Three: Identify Current Path

Connect all of the boxes selected for the current approach to each dimension. This path is the current market stance.

Step Four: Identify a New Path

Connect all of the boxes selected for the preferred approach to each dimension. This new path describes the preferred market stance.

Step Five: Develop Preferred Market Stance

Once each participant has identified his or her preferred path, the planning group should discuss as a whole each dimension and agree on a preferred fundamental approach for the organization.

Working as a group, the planning committee should:

1. Articulate a preferred new path or market stance by "connecting the boxes."
2. Establish a qualitative and quantitative rationale for the preferred path, based upon the foundation established in phases one and two.
3. Agree on how the new path differs from today's path or stance.
4. Identify the major implications of the new path.

Step Six: Formulate Goals

For each dimension of the game, formulate a major goal statement that articulates the overall objectives that the organization is trying to achieve along the dimension. For example, in Figure 6.1, the organization's goal for column A, horizontal integration, might read "Expand the continuum of care through collaborative arrangements with area providers and physicians." The goal for column E, geographic focus, might be to "Expand system market share in outlying portions of the service area."

Step Seven: Identify Strategies

For each dimension of the game, particularly where the current path diverges from the preferred path, develop strategies that help the organization achieve its goals. Identifying strategies and developing measures of success are described fully in the next chapter.

Figure 6.1. The New Path.

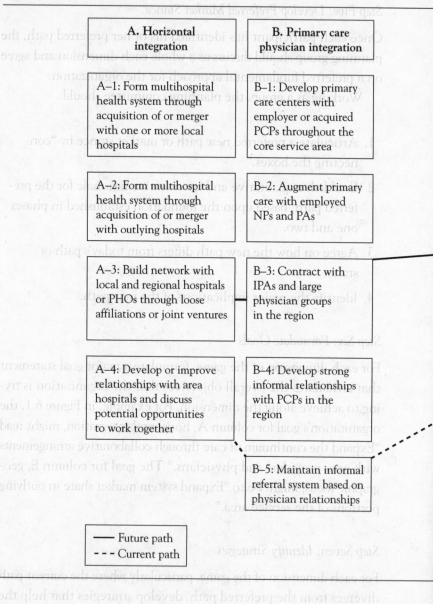

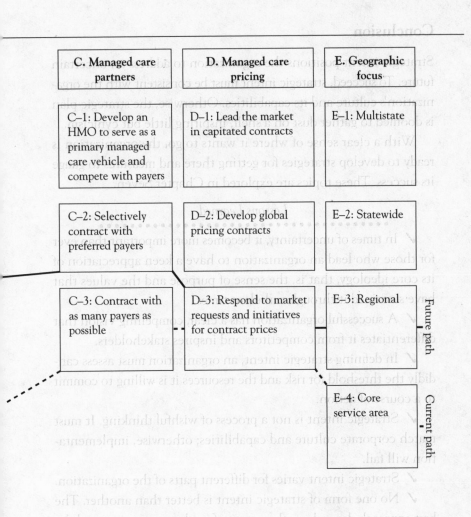

Conclusion

Strategic intent positions the organization to address an uncertain future. To succeed, strategic intent must be consistent with the organization's culture and its capabilities. Otherwise, the strategic plan is doomed to gather dust on a shelf, inspiring little but cynicism.

With a clear sense of where it wants to go, the organization is ready to develop strategies for getting there and measures to gauge its success. These topics are explored in Chapter Seven.

Lessons Learned

✓ In times of uncertainty, it becomes more important than ever for those who lead an organization to have a keen appreciation of its core ideology, that is, the sense of purpose and the values that have sustained it through turbulent times.

✓ A successful organization has a clear, compelling vision that differentiates it from competitors and inspires stakeholders.

✓ In defining strategic intent, an organization must assess candidly the threshold for risk and the resources it is willing to commit to a course of action.

✓ Strategic intent is not a process of wishful thinking. It must match corporate culture and capabilities; otherwise, implementation will fail.

✓ Strategic intent varies for different parts of the organization.

✓ No one form of strategic intent is better than another. The best approach depends on the extent of market uncertainty and the characteristics of the organization.

Developing Strategies
and Measures of Success

Thomas R. Miller and Elizabeth S. Bashore

With so much uncertainty in the environment, how can an organization develop effective strategies? Once developed, what can the organization do to assess the progress of these strategies? How does the organization monitor market changes and determine whether adjustments are needed to its planning assumptions?

As described in Chapter Six, an organization's core ideology, vision, and market stance define its strategic intent. Developing strategies and **measures of success** builds upon strategic intent and constitutes phase four of the strategy cycle (see Figure 2.3). This chapter examines formulation of types of strategy and measures of success based on the organization's strategic intent; it includes guidelines for developing them in an increasingly uncertain environment.

Importance of Strategy and
Measures of Success Development

Although strategies and measures of success are integral components of traditional strategic planning, they become highly important in an era of uncertainty. In a stable environment, there is tolerance for error, and organizations have the ability to recover if they make mistakes. In an unstable environment, however, organizations must be able to conduct interim measurements in the course of long-term strategies to make critical adjustments to them. In addition, they must monitor the external environment or market to determine when to change the planning assumptions associated with those strategies.

Strategies are courses of action representing the "how" to achieve the "what" of an organization's strategic intent. Strategies also have been defined as "the basic characteristics of the match an organization achieves with its environment" (Hofer and Schendel, 1978, p. 4). This definition emphasizes the importance of developing strategies that reflect the environmental assessment and leadership's planning assumptions, as well as describing how the organization's strategic intent is to be achieved. Strategy development is the culmination of the strategic planning process; as such, it can be the most challenging aspect.

Measures of success are, collectively, a benchmark to monitor an organization's progress toward successful implementation of its strategic intent and specific strategies. Measures of success also enable an organization to test the validity of its planning assumptions. Measures include both "metrics" and "triggers."

Metrics are internal indicators that monitor the organization's short-term performance related to implementing its long-term strategies. Metrics are internal measures in that they gauge an organization's success or failure in implementing strategies. However, metrics can be external or internal, depending on whether the organization's strategies focus on the larger market or internally. For example, external metrics include an organization's market share, relative cost position in the market, and performance against benchmark quality indicators. They reflect organization-specific performance, albeit against marketwide data. Thresholds of acceptable performance provide target levels that, if not met during strategy implementation, generally indicate a need for management intervention and action. Although metrics can be both a subset of and a supplement to the dashboard of key indicators that hospitals and health systems use to monitor the overall health of the organization, this chapter discusses metrics as they relate to specific strategies.

Triggers, by contrast, are external indicators that enable the organization to monitor overall market changes and test the validity of its planning assumptions. Organizations must know when their planning assumptions are no longer reasonable since changes in planning assumptions may indicate the need to change strategies. It is critical to use both metrics and triggers to achieve expected performance levels. These measures are discussed in detail later in this chapter.

Impacts of Strategic Intent, Uncertainty, and Strategies

Both the strategic intent of an organization and the level of uncertainty in its environment influence the development of strategies and their associated measures of success. To overcome the inertia that uncertainty can produce, it is imperative that leaders develop clear, focused strategies to compensate for a seemingly unclear and unfocused environment.

Table 7.1 summarizes the major implications of strategic intent and uncertainty for developing strategies. Although the three prototypes of strategic intent—the market enactor, the market adapter, and the market survivor—are illustrated, it is important to remember that an organization's strategic intent is not always exclusively one behavior. An organization that is a market survivor overall could have a big-bet strategy for one of its service lines.

As an example, in 1997, Sinai Hospital of Baltimore employed what we would consider a big-bet strategy for a service line by renovating its emergency department to include seven distinct care centers: fast-track, urgent, emergent, pediatric, trauma, observation, and a special chest pain evaluation center (Voelker, 1999). ER-7, as the project was called, was implemented in the face of managed care, where emphasis is placed on controlling emergency room use, admissions, and inappropriate access points for care. Contrary to popular belief, Sinai Hospital believed that there was a need for customer service in the emergency department and that the emergency

Table 7.1. Strategic-Development Implications
of Strategic Intent and Uncertainty.

Strategic Intent	General Characteristics of Strategies	Implications of Increasing Uncertainty for Strategy Development
Market enactor	Focus on market position Substantial in nature High-risk (big bets) Significant changes targeted Longer implementation time	No fundamental changes Increased need for communications within the organization regarding strategic intent and rationale (planning assumptions and environmental assessment) Externally focused metrics
Market adapter	Both market and internal focus Strategies that are popular, less disruptive, and easily changed Incremental changes targeted Generally shorter implementation time	Copycat strategies Increased schizophrenia and pluralistic approaches Less willing to commit significant resources

Market survivor	Internally focused
	  Quality
	  Cost
	  Customer service
		Strategic intent chosen by majority of organizations
		Less willing to commit significant resources to strategies
		Organization must still watch for market opportunities to decide when to make a strategic move

department could be used as a marketing tool. Warren Green, president and chief executive officer of Lifebridge Health, parent company of Sinai Hospital of Baltimore, stated the "field of dreams" perspective: "If you develop a better product, people will come." As a result of its strategy, patient satisfaction survey results improved and emergency department visits increased from 54,000 in 1996 to about 70,000 per year in subsequent years. Although Sinai Hospital could have another strategic intent overall, it successfully implemented a market-enactor strategy at the level of emergency services.

The impacts of strategic intent and uncertainty on developing strategies and metrics, the internal measures, are described fully below. External triggers are revisited later in the chapter.

Strategies and Metrics of Market Enactors

Market enactors are rare in any industry, and rarer still in health care. As described in Table 7.1, enactors seek not only to establish a leading market position but to change the market. They choose risky strategies, or big-bet approaches, that can create big payoffs but that also carry significant downside risk. In general, market enactors do not alter their fundamental vision in an environment of uncertainty; rather, they see uncertainty as facilitating opportunities to define and shape the environment in which they compete and operate.

Strategy development for the market enactor should be leadership-driven and have single-minded focus. Leaders in a true market enactor organization ride out small setbacks and failures, thanks to the expectation that it will win the big bet in the long run.

Although uncertainty does not change the strategy of market enactors, it increases the need for effective internal communication of the organization's strategic intent. In addition, substantial constituency education is needed regarding the rationale underlying the organization's vision. The need to create structure to deal with uncertainty in the environment and to educate board members, employees, and affiliated physicians reinforces the case for diligence, rigor, and focus in developing the environmental assessment and planning assumptions.

Table 7.2 gives examples of strategies for each type of strategic intent around four major strategic areas relevant to one hospital system. The areas, a subset of those identified through the new-path exercise discussed at the end of Chapter Six, are horizontal integration, primary care physician integration, managed care partners, and managed care pricing. In general, high-risk strategies are associated with market enactors. In our example, representative big-bet strategies include forming a multihospital health system through acquisition or merger with one or more local hospitals; developing primary care centers with employed or acquired physicians throughout the core service area; developing an HMO; and significantly expanding the capitated contracts with which the hospital participates. Given that their intent is to fundamentally change the market, it is not surprising that these strategies are not as widespread in popularity and have fewer demonstrated successes.

The metrics employed by market enactors also focus on the structure of the market and the market position of the organization. Table 7.3 has examples of metrics relevant to the three prototypes of strategic intent. For market enactors, examples of metrics are market share, the percentage of primary care physicians affiliated with the system, and the hospital's or system's percentage of the total market enrolled lives.

Market enactors establish targets that reflect their expectations of significant changes in these metrics as a result of their big-bet moves. For example, targeted market share increases of 25–50 percent are not uncommon.

Strategies and Metrics of Market Adapters

As shown in Table 7.1, strategies of market adapters respond to the characteristics of the market and often reflect popular strategies that can be found in markets across the country. Like the market enactor, market adapters have a clear vision but are less likely to expend considerable resources until the market trends become clear

Table 7.2. Examples of Hospital "New Path" Strategies Based on Strategic Intent.

Strategic Intent	Examples of Strategies Within Selected Strategic Areas			
	Horizontal Integration	Primary Care Physician Integration	Managed Care Partners	Managed Care Pricing
Market enactor	A–1: Form multihospital health system through acquisition of or merger with one or more local hospitals	B–1: Develop primary care centers with employed or acquired PCPs throughout the core service area	C–1: Develop an HMO to serve as a primary managed care vehicle and compete with payers	D–1: Lead the market in capitated contracts
Market adapter	A–3: Build network with local and regional hospitals or PHOs through loose affiliations or joint ventures	B–3: Contract with IPAs and large physician groups in the region	C–2: Selectively contract with preferred payers	D–2: Develop global pricing contracts
Market survivor	A–4: Develop or improve relationships with area hospitals and discuss potential opportunities to work together	B–4: Develop strong informal relationships with PCPs in the region	C–3: Contract with as many payers as possible	D–3: Respond to market requests and initiatives for contract prices

Table 7.3. Examples of Metrics Based on Strategic Intent.

Strategic Intent	Examples of Metrics
Market enactor	Market share
	Affiliated primary care physicians as percentage of market
	Percentage of total market enrolled lives
Market adapter	Change in market share
	Financial performance
	Quality indicators
	Industry benchmarks
Market survivor	Financial performance
	Quality indicators
	Results of customer service surveys:
	Employee
	Patient
	Physician
	Area consumers

and the likelihood of success with a strategy is great. Internally oriented initiatives become important as they are necessary to change the organization's structure and processes to effectively meet the needs of external customers and payers and to respond to competitor initiatives.

Market adapters tend to follow rather than lead market change, often behaving like copycats. Although adapters are less innovative in choosing which strategies to adopt, successful market adapters innovate and excel in how they implement those strategies. However, in formulating strategies, adapters can fall into the trap of trying to identify and pursue strategies that have already worked for similar organizations in similar markets. Such "twins," though, rarely exist. Even small differences in the dynamics of two markets or organizations can result in large variation in the success of a strategy. Additionally, even if twins do exist, many organizations do not recognize their twin because they have not done an adequate job of objectively describing themselves and their markets in developing the environmental assessment.

In uncertain times, health care leaders stress the need to be flexible. Flexibility is seen as a positive trait in today's unstable environment since it allows the organization to minimize risk because it can quickly adjust its path. Though an attractive principle, flexibility is occasionally a reflection of leadership's unwillingness or inability to commit to a specific course for the organization. For example, during the keynote address at a recent planning retreat of a large regional health system, this is how the CEO articulated the system's strategy: "We are employing a pluralistic approach to physician integration in recognition of the unique markets in which we operate." At a subsequent after-dinner setting, the CEO admitted to a few individuals that "we really have no idea what to do and are trying anything and everything in hopes that something works." In contrast, a market enactor has a clear preference regarding its approach to physician integration, regardless of how integration actually may be implemented in a particular market.

As indicated in Table 7.2, strategies for market adapters are being implemented simultaneously in many markets. They are less big-bet oriented and therefore safer for the organization if major environmental changes occur. Examples of such strategies include developing a network with local providers through loose affiliations, contracting with large physician groups or contracting entities in the region, and developing some moderately risky global pricing contracts with preferred payers. These strategies lend room for change if the need occurs because there is lower investment, less risk, and more flexibility.

Market adapters use market and internal metrics; in particular they look to benchmarks and comparison with similar organizations in similar markets. As indicated in Table 7.3, typical metrics include market share and market share growth, cost and quality comparisons by specialty or diagnosis, and financial performance related to managed care plans or service lines. Compared to market enactors, market adapters target relatively small changes in these metrics.

As uncertainty increases, market adapters may develop a need to compare more and more performance metrics with other organizations. This type of comparison can be beneficial because it allows the organization to measure itself with others that may be the best of the best, therefore encouraging improvement and innovation in operational and financial processes. However, if not done within this context of improvement and innovation, these comparisons can bestow a false sense of security. For example, hospital leaders may find it acceptable to incur substantial losses on a physician network development strategy if "everyone else is losing money also."

Strategies and Metrics of Market Survivors

In an environment of uncertainty, many organizations prepare for action but make few strategic moves. Strategies become internally focused, often around work redesign, quality enhancement, and cost reduction. Although these initiatives have merit for internal improvements, they are not effective substitutes for strategy regarding an organization's product offerings, customers, potential partners, and market position. In contrast, many market survivors avoid severe headaches by taking a wait-and-see approach, particularly in the areas of physician practice acquisitions and large-scale capitation arrangements.

Many health care organizations have tremendous opportunities to improve their efficiency and effectiveness in the areas of service, cost, and quality. An internally focused strategic plan often seems successful because of the substantial operational improvements that can be made. It does not take long, however, for organizations that are too internally focused to grow out of touch with the market and dig a competitive hole from which they may not recover. Therefore, market survivors too must continuously assess opportunities in the market to determine whether and when to make a strategic move.

As presented in the examples in Table 7.2, market survivors (or health care organizations that are "reserving the right to play") view participation in an alliance or collaborative discussions with other providers as appropriate horizontal integration strategies. Managed care strategies for these organizations may focus on maintaining flexibility in accepting contract partners and prices in order to play with as many as possible. Physician integration strategies are rarely action-oriented, instead focusing on enhancing physician relationships through improving communication; offering physicians greater opportunities to participate in leadership; providing support services such as marketing and information systems; and improving physician-related customer service by facilitating surgery and ancillary scheduling, offering better parking and dining areas, and enhancing physician work and rest areas.

Typically, metrics for market survivor organizations are consistent with their strategic initiatives and are internally focused. As indicated in Table 7.3, they generally include an array of financial, quality, and customer service indicators that become the basis for promoting the organization's strengths and attracting potential partners with which to play.

Validity of Planning Assumptions

In implementing a strategy, an organization might not succeed for four basic reasons:

1. The organization lacks the financial capability to fully implement the strategy.

2. The strategy is not implemented correctly, or perhaps not at all.

3. The culture of the organization creates insurmountable obstacles to implementation.

4. The strategy is based on planning assumptions that are no longer valid.

The financial causes of failure to implement are discussed further in Chapter Eight. The organizational challenges that cause implementation to be stalled or ineffective are the focus of Chapter Nine. In this section, we focus on the fourth basic reason; that is, the planning assumptions are no longer valid.

As explained previously, triggers alert an organization to significant changes in the overall market. Because the underlying planning assumptions build upon the environmental assessment, these market changes may require that the planning assumptions be adjusted and strategies changed to reflect new trends or practices in the market.

Various environmental triggers challenge an organization's strategies, depending on its strategic intent. An organization that strives to lead the market in capitated contracts, a representative strategy of a market enactor, may discover that this strategy needs to be adjusted or changed if the number of covered lives in the market declines or strong public sentiment increases around having a choice in providers. The market adapter that plans to build networks through loose affiliations may need an aggressive approach if its two largest competitors merge. The market survivor seeking contracts with as many payers as possible in an attempt to reserve the right to play may question its strategy if it finds that the number of exclusive contracts between payers and its competitors is increasing significantly.

Each of these triggers significantly changes the market assumptions on which the strategies are based. No matter how effectively or efficiently the strategy is implemented, the organization will not achieve success because the market has shifted. Therefore, it is absolutely critical that the organization incorporate triggers in its measurement process to limit unnecessary frustration and resource expenditures.

Knowledge of Strategic Intent Is Not Enough

Although strategic intent helps define an organization's strategies and measures of success, it is merely a starting point. Developing strategies requires hard work, a thorough planning process, candid dialogue, appropriate analyses, and commitment of resources to the process. In an era of uncertainty, organizations are susceptible to the pitfalls that commonly arise in strategy development. The sections that follow present a few overarching principles and guidelines to improve an organization's effectiveness in developing strategies and measures of success.

Importance of Strategic Clarity and Focus

Developing a strategic plan is both a process and a product. The process has been described earlier in this book. Uncertainty increases the need for an approach that is leadership-driven and founded on a solid base of information regarding the internal and external environment and expected trends.

The product includes strategy statements, whose meanings and subsequent implementation are, to a great extent, dependent on the language chosen by the leadership team. In an environment of uncertainty, organizations that develop generic or broad strategies simply compound the uncertainty and create an unnecessary hurdle to acceptance of the strategies by the management team and others responsible for implementation.

Strategies should be both meaningful and significant. In an uncertain environment, leaders may be tempted to develop a plan that includes watered-down strategies lacking specificity and decisiveness. The desire to achieve consensus in a planning group often drives the temptation to develop diluted strategies. This tendency may be reinforced by a perverse sense of required political correctness, or a misguided attempt at equality among all products or customers. For example, it is often difficult for hospital leaders to establish orthopedics as a center of excellence if that might imply that urology is not.

Strategies should reflect trade-offs and priority setting. As discussed in Chapter Six in the section on creating a new path, a sustainable strategic position requires trade-offs that create the need for choice and purposely limit what a company offers (Porter, 1996).

These tasks of selection become difficult in an uncertain environment. Market adapters faced with great uncertainty are often compelled to entertain all potential strategies with equal fervor. They can become paralyzed and unable to make effective or timely decisions. This paralysis contradicts the market adapter's desire to be flexible and responsive.

How can priority setting and decisions involving trade-offs become more acceptable to an organization? Developing appropriate base information in the environmental assessment, planning with clear assumptions, and understanding an organization's financial and human resource capacity are all vital in helping support a specific direction or strategy that may seem, on the surface, to exclude other important organizational initiatives.

Strategies alone are the mechanism for achieving the organization's goals. However, once strategies are developed, the organization must begin to focus on effective implementation and measurement of performance related to those strategies. Measures of success should be used to add substance to the strategy statements and give direction in their implementation.

Guidelines for Developing Measures of Success

Measures of success should be developed primarily to assess an organization's objectives for and progress in implementing its strategies. Although not every strategy requires a unique set of measures, the identified measures should help monitor progress on most of the organization's strategies. To increase the effectiveness of performance measurement, organizations should use certain basic guidelines in developing measures of success, as the next sections suggest.

Develop Corridors of Acceptable Values for Metrics

Corridors or parameters of acceptable values should be developed in conjunction with metrics to alert management of underperformance early in the process, before considerable time, effort, and resources have been invested in an initiative. If strategies cover a two-to three-year time frame, each metric should be monitored quarterly or every six months to ensure that it falls within the acceptable corridor and, if not, that appropriate actions have been identified and taken. At the very least, metrics should be monitored annually, whether the organization is a market enactor or a market survivor.

For example, suppose management targets a certain level for the number of covered lives associated with the hospital's PHO for the next two years. The number of covered lives could be reviewed quarterly, or monthly calculated on a three-month moving average. Management would consider a significant change of course or intervention only if the three-month average number of covered lives reaches a preestablished threshold of, say, 30 percent below the target.

Identify Triggers Up Front

Environmental triggers should be identified as planning assumptions are developed and, if scenario planning is used, when alternative futures are articulated. Identifying triggers up front encourages the organization to consider how the market may change. For example, if an organization's strategy is to develop an open-heart surgery service, which external triggers indicate that the strategy is not a good one? The planning assumptions include a projected significant increase in the population over sixty-five years of age and a continued strong relationship between the hospital and a large multispecialty physician practice that includes high-volume cardiac surgeons. If the population increase fails to materialize or a competitor acquires the multispecialty group, does this strategy still make sense? Triggers are valuable because they indicate whether the organization needs to reevaluate its core strategies and associated assumptions.

Ensure That Measures Are Clear and Data Are Available

Every management team member should clearly understand each measure of success and the basis for its measurement. A measure of success, including either metrics or triggers, is useful to the organization only if data are available with which to compare actual and targeted results. The organization must ensure that information is available to the person or group assigned to the task of measurement, and that the process and technology are in place to gather the appropriate information. It is not necessary that all of the information be available within the organization, but how and where to obtain outside data must be clearly defined.

Although the third guideline is a seemingly simple principle, failing to take data availability into account is a trap into which organizations that are developing formal measures for the first time often fall. Here are examples of metrics identified by hospitals and subsequently discarded from lack of information availability or systems to simplify data collection:

- Number of patients that would not have come to the hospital if the ambulatory strategy had not been implemented

- Profitability of outpatient pediatric services

- Percentage of total admissions of employees from ABC Manufacturing Co.

- Quality of physical therapy services compared to area competitors

Assign Accountability for Metrics, and Incorporate Them into Performance Objectives

A person or group must be accountable to the measurement process if it is to occur on schedule and correctly. Depending on the scope of the metrics, there are a number of people within the organization who could share this responsibility, and each of these individuals may bring his or her own perspective to the initiative. For instance, assigning the responsibility to senior management lends importance and visibility to the initiative. Assigning the responsibility to a group that is accustomed to measuring performance lends experience to the initiative. Assigning it to a group that has no experience in performance measurement increases exposure and learning.

Once metrics have been identified, selected targets should be incorporated into the objectives and performance evaluations of senior and midlevel managers who have the appropriate level of authority to oversee initiatives and authorize corrective action. This process links performance to compensation and motivates the manager to focus on personal goals and strategies that are critical to the organization's long-term success. Linking rewards to performance, however, is effective only if the individual has substantial control over the outcomes that he or she is responsible for achieving.

Develop a Balanced Set of Metrics

Develop a **balanced scorecard** of metrics that incorporate but go beyond the traditional financial indicators. As discussed in Chapter Three, many organizations are implementing a dashboard of key indicators, which encourages the organization to focus on key financial, operational, quality, and other performance indicators across the organization.

The Balanced Scorecard

In the early 1990s, the balanced scorecard was developed as a tool in corporate industry to link an organization's financial indicators to measurement in three other areas: customers, internal business processes, and learning and growth (Kaplan and Norton, 1996b). What was originally intended as a tool for monitoring these four perspectives became a strategic management system used by organizations of all types and sizes. The tool is not meant to supplant financial metrics but instead to complement them with metrics from other areas that contribute to the long-term success of the organization. In short, the process links short-term actions and long-term strategy implementation.

In health care, measuring financial results is certainly critical to the organization if it is to remain in business, particularly with declining payments and growing concern about providing health care coverage to all people. However, especially in a not-for-profit organization, long-term success goes beyond financial metrics. If only financial performance were measured, the organization could acquire a distorted view of its performance. For example, strong financial results for a hospital in the last quarter of the fiscal year may have occurred at the expense of patient satisfaction thanks to staff shortages during periods of extremely high census levels.

In our experience, the original balanced scorecard perspectives are easily adapted for the not-for-profit health care organization to include ownership, market, internal business processes, and innovation, all of which are critical to long-term success. To examine itself and its strategies holistically, the organization must ask itself these questions:

- How do we meet the needs of our owners, that is, the community or the religious sponsors?

- As not-for-profit providers, how do we invest in the community?

- How do we meet the needs of patients, physicians, and payers?

- In which processes must we excel so as to thrive and remain competitive?

- How can we continue to grow as an innovative, learning organization?

As metrics within each of these perspectives begin to overlap, the organization naturally develops its dashboard of key indicators. An explanation of the four balanced perspectives for health care

Table 7.4. Four Common Organizational Perspectives.

Perspective	Answers the Question:	Focuses on:
Ownership	How does the organization meet the needs of its owners? How does it invest in the community that it serves?	Community benefit, community health, profitability, value
Market	How does the organization meet the needs of its customers, including patients, physicians, payers, etc.?	Value, performance, service
Internal business processes	What processes must the organization do well in to thrive and remain competitive?	Technology, people, processes, quality
Innovation	How can the organization continue to grow as an innovative, learning organization?	People, systems, processes

Source: Adapted from Kaplan and Norton (1996b).

organizations and the focus of associated metrics is included in Table 7.4.

Table 7.5 presents potential metrics related to a health system's ambulatory care strategy using a balanced scorecard approach. Depending on the market characteristics, the organization portrayed could be either a market enactor or a market adapter. At the strategy level, both organization types employ similar metrics. For example, metrics relating to a physician-friendly environment and patient origin analyses help to examine the uncertainty regarding physician loyalty and use of satellite ambulatory care facilities versus hospital-based services. Table 7.5 also illustrates the relationships and interdependencies among the four balanced scorecard perspectives and the potential metrics.

Table 7.5. A Balanced Approach to Developing Metrics for a Hospital's Ambulatory Care Strategy.

Strategy: Provide geographically distributed health services by developing major ambulatory care sites, including at least two with ambulatory surgery services.

Uncertainty	Implication	Potential Metrics	Perspective
How will physician loyalty change? Will they use the ambulatory site or continue to use hospital-based services?	Must make new sites efficient and easy to use for physicians	Incremental volume by service (based on total volume at ambulatory sites and hospital campus)	Ownership
		Percentage of patients from targeted or underserved geographic areas	Ownership
		Percentage of time that key physicians get first or second choice for operating room times	Market
		Billing cycle time	Internal processes
		Degree to which staff understands and uses billing and scheduling systems	Internal processes
		Cannibalization of hospital-based services	Ownership

Question	Statement	Measure	Category
How will competitors respond? Will they develop their own ambulatory care sites?	Must build strong relationships with patients and physicians and respond to market needs for services	Number of preventive health classes provided to community	Ownership
		Physician satisfaction surveys	Market
		Patient satisfaction surveys	Market
		Patient referrals within system versus outside of system	Ownership
		Number and time frame for introduction of new services and programs	Innovation
		Scheduling flexibility	Internal processes
Will managed care plans contract with the new sites long-term? For which services? At what rates?	Must provide value-added services	Cost per procedure or visit	Ownership
		Covered lives by payer	Ownership
		Billing cycle time	Internal processes
		Market share by payer	Ownership
		Contribution margin	Ownership
		Visits and procedures by physicians and physician extenders	Internal processes
		Patient satisfaction	Market

Conclusion

This chapter has discussed strategies and measures of success and how their development is affected by strategic intent and uncertainty. Strategies and measures of success are traditional planning components and tools that are more important than ever in this era of uncertainty. Because there is little room for error in an unstable environment, health care organizations must be able to assess short-term performance relative to long-term strategies, be aware of market triggers, and quickly make adjustments before substantial resources are committed or competitors take advantage of market opportunities. Once strategies are identified, the organization must ensure it has sufficient financial capability and the appropriate culture, structure, and processes in place to ensure success in implementation. These topics are discussed in the following two chapters.

Lessons Learned

✓ Strategies and measures of success reflect an organization's strategic intent coupled with the level of uncertainty in the environment.

✓ Strategy development and measures of success build upon information developed in the environmental assessment and the planning assumptions.

✓ Measures of success include the internal measures (metrics) that are used to assess performance related to a particular strategy, and the external measures (triggers) that alert the organization to potential changes in a strategy's underlying planning assumptions. Both are critical to achieving long-term success.

✓ Identifying priorities among strategies and making trade-offs are both difficult in an era of uncertainty. However, lack of such decisiveness and commitment simply increases the organization's level of uncertainty.

✓ Senior managers must lead the strategy development process and be held accountable for successful implementation.

✓ Uncertainty shortens the relevant planning time frame. Metrics can be used to perform short-term assessments of long-term strategies.

✓ A balanced approach should be taken in developing metrics, to augment financial indicators with others that relate to the organization's core ideology and preferred market stance.

✓ Measures of success should be meaningful, easily understood, and monitored.

8

Financial Planning in an Era of Uncertainty

J. Bruce Ryan and Judith E. Belt

Does a strategy exist if resources are not available to make it happen? Can financial and strategic planning be separated? Strategic planning is, de facto, a process to allocate scarce resources. The true reflection of strategic priorities is not a written plan; rather, it is the manner in which an organization chooses to invest its capital. Ignoring financial planning as an integral part of overall strategic planning is tantamount to relying on luck to secure an organization's future. Although financial planning is a dynamic process, it requires a structured approach to ensure that the organization makes the best strategic decisions, based on its objectives and projected financial resources.

Financial planning includes three key components, which form the basis for this chapter:

1. Assessing financial capability. Review the organization's ability to generate capital over the planning horizon.

2. Evaluating alternative uses. Determine the organization's needs and the relative risks of alternatives.

3. Allocating resources. Distribute the organization's financial capability by earmarking funds for the various strategic alternatives, and develop decision rules on how to fund and allocate the financial capability.

The Challenges of
Financial Planning Amid Uncertainty

One of the uncontested facts of life is that financial demands exceed available resources. There are few exceptions to this rule, whether on the personal side (from how to spend an allowance as a child to determining how much of a house you can afford as an adult) or the business side (where no organization can afford to do everything). However, the inevitable mismatch between desired uses and available sources of funds assumes even greater significance given the high level of uncertainty about the future of health care and continued pressures on cash flows. As discussed in Chapter One, the number of strategic alternatives available to health care organizations is significantly greater than in the past, the environment in which organizations will exist is outside of anyone's domain of experience, the exact actions necessary to succeed in the new environment are not known, and speculation may rise to the level of a primary decision tool.

As noted in Chapter Six, financial planning is critically important regardless of the form of strategic intent (market enactor, market adapter, or market survivor). Strategic intent may determine the magnitude of needed financial resources and allocation of them. For instance, a market enactor must have an extremely strong financial position to initiate and sustain its strategies, while a market adapter typically requires fewer financial resources but needs enough financial capability to redirect funds to respond to market opportunities. A market survivor must have sufficient resources to stay in the game.

Then again, available financial resources may drive strategic intent. For example, it would be difficult for an organization with limited financial capability to adopt a market-enactor approach, and organizations with significant capital resources may be missing tremendous opportunity by seeking only to survive the shakeout.

At its most basic, financial planning can be characterized as a balancing act that seeks to reconcile financial capability and strategic direction; the interests of diverse constituencies, including the trustees, management, physicians, and the local community; mission and vision, short-term financial feasibility, and long-term financial success; and the risks and potential rewards of alternative directions.

The balancing act becomes considerably more difficult and complex in an era of uncertainty, when, simultaneously, the number of alternative directions increases, availability of funds is reduced, and decisions are perceived to be riskier than during an era of stability. CFO magazine identifies health care as one of the most difficult industries for financial decision making and contends that healthcare CFOs have "served as scapegoats for a flailing industry" (McCafferty, 1999, p. 64).

There have been major financial failures and disappointments across the health care continuum in the last few years, resulting from not fully anticipating or managing uncertainty. These include financial failures (see Table 8.1), as well as significant losses incurred

Table 8.1. Financial Failures Across the Health Care Continuum.

Industry Segment	Company	Bankruptcy or Insolvency Date
Hospital systems	Allegheny Health Education and Research Foundation (AHERF; Hensley, 1998)	July 1998
Physician practice management	FPA Medical Management (Jaklevic, 1998)	July 1998
Health maintenance organizations	HIP Health Plans of New Jersey (McCarthy, 1999)	February 1999
Home health	Home Health Corporations of America ("News at Deadline . . . ," 1999)	February 1999
Long-term care	NewCare Health Corp. ("For the Record . . . ," 1999b)	June 1999

by provider-owned HMOs and hospital-owned physician practices. The financial losses sustained from acquired physician practices are not surprising since this strategy was primarily a defensive move, one often made without consideration of the long-term financial implications.

According to a Moody's press release, we can "expect more bankruptcy filings to occur as hospitals are unable to make bond payments and seek relief from creditors" (Goldstein, 1999, p. 34). These failures and the increasingly uncertain health care environment are decreasing the ratings of hospital debt, which in turn are increasing the cost and decreasing the availability of credit. Until providers learn how to operate in this environment, their financial future will remain bleak.

Planning for the future must be based on the best information currently available and on the organization's resource availability, current and forecast. It is natural to feel uncomfortable allocating resources to the moving target of the future health care environment. However, uncertainty can result in an organization's management focusing on the wrong issues. Just as the railroads floundered by defining themselves as railroad companies instead of transportation companies, hospitals could experience the same type of decline if they misread the uncertain future and develop poorly focused strategies. To avoid the same fate as the railroad industry, financial planning must be an integral component of health care strategic planning. All parties involved must be comfortable with financial planning since it offers insight into the decision-making process under uncertainty, thus ensuring the long-term economic viability of the organization.

Assess Financial Capability

A simple definition of *financial capability* is the amount of capital, both debt and investments, that a health care organization can generate to invest while safely maintaining its operations. Capital is generated from five sources: current liquid asset balances, cash flow generated from future operations, philanthropy, new debt, and infusions of equity capital. Although there might be potential for a nonprofit organization to raise equity capital for certain for-profit activities, given the recent poor performance of health care equities in the capital market this source is not discussed in this chapter. We briefly discuss the other four sources and the inherent uncertainties in each.

Current Liquid Asset Balances

Liquid assets are cash or those assets that can quickly be converted to cash. This component of financial capability is the simplest to calculate but is mired in the politics of the organization. The issue affecting financial capability is how much of the current reserves the organization is willing to risk. These reserves are typically what allow board members and management to sleep well. However, the ability to maintain these reserves in the future is uncertain.

Cash Flow Generated from Future Operations

Cash flow generated from future operations represents the projected financial performance of the existing or future business. This component of financial capacity is undoubtedly the most volatile and has significant impact on the other components. The 1997 Balanced Budget Act and unfavorable managed care contracts have significantly and negatively affected most health care organizations, including hospitals, home health, and nursing homes, and they continue to weaken financial capability.

Nationwide, hospital operating margins dropped 45 percent in the fourth quarter of 1998 compared with 1997 (Moore, 1999a). Many hospitals have propped up sagging operating margins with returns from investment of reserves. However, the unpredictability of the financial markets and the growing need to dip into those reserves for both operations and strategic initiatives is likely to hurt this source of bottom-line profitability. During these volatile times, applying historical trends to predict future financial outcomes is not a prudent exercise; bottom-line growth is no longer a safe bet.

Philanthropy

Philanthropy is becoming an increasingly important, albeit unpredictable, source of financial capability, as evidenced by the $16.9 billion raised by health organizations in 1998, a 20.4 percent increase over 1997 ("For the Record . . . ," 1999a). As Clark Bell noted in an editorial in *Modern Healthcare,* "Donations, grants and wise investment decisions will help determine on which side of the profit ledger your organization falls" (1999, p. 32).

New Debt

The incremental amount of debt an organization can assume at a targeted level of risk is known as debt capacity. This can be measured in one of two ways: a balance sheet approach or a cash-flow approach. Under the balance sheet approach, ratios (such as debts to assets) are used to determine the upper limit of the organization's ability to carry debt. In the cash-flow approach, the amount of debt is measured by determining how much debt the organization can afford to repay based on its cash flows.

Calculating and using an organization's debt capacity hinges on many variables, some of which are controllable and others are not. For instance, interest rates are beyond the control of hospitals since a single hospital or industry does not influence fluctuations in the financial market. However, organizational risk preferences and investment and consumption decisions are within the organization's control. Each organization has a certain debt capacity, but organizations have differing positions on using it. For instance, an aggressive health care company may choose to use 80 percent of its debt capacity, while another hospital may choose to borrow only 40 percent of its capacity.

It is important to remember that debt capacity is dynamic, and each strategic decision changes the debt capacity of the organization and has an impact on the funds available for other strategic initiatives. For instance, if a hospital acquires a long-term care facility for $20 million, the impact on the debt capacity for other strategic initiatives is not limited to this initial purchase price. The impact also includes, say, $2 million required for renovation, and funding losses for the first three years of operations of another $3 million. Therefore, debt capacity available to finance other strategic initiatives is reduced by $25 million.

Evaluate Alternative Uses

As previously mentioned, the demand for capital is unlimited. The traditional approach to financial planning, which includes selecting from a limited number of alternatives (taking into account the level of risk the organization is willing and able to assume), is still appropriate during times of uncertainty. The challenge during times of change is to evaluate the relative risks of alternative strategies.

Assessing and Managing Risk

In an era of uncertainty, assessing and managing the risks of alternative strategies is one of the most important functions of the financial team. As pointed out in a recent *Healthcare Financial Management* article, "For many healthcare organizations, the pursuit of popular strategies based on commonly held perceptions of the healthcare environment has led to difficulties because financial decision makers did not adequately account for the risks associated with those strategies" (Kleinmuntz, Kleinmuntz, Stephen, and Nordlund, 1999, p. 51).

Identifying the true risk of future events requires stripping away the layers of uncertainty in the current environment. Although it is not reasonable to expect that uncertainty can be eliminated, there are some basic steps that can be taken to assess the magnitude of the risk, if not the underlying risk distribution. Chapter Five contains a thorough discussion of tools commonly used to address uncertainty, including scenario planning and decision analysis. These tools are used extensively in financial planning and help organizations focus attention on facts that are likely to have a material impact on the future, as well as to eliminate strategies that have low likelihood of success.

Health care organizations must keep in mind that "the reasons a strategy failed often are clear in hindsight. The challenge is to understand and anticipate risk in a way that promotes optimum success, before launching the initiative" (Kleinmuntz, Kleinmuntz, Stephen, and Nordlund, 1999, p. 51). It is important to be aware of common pitfalls in the quest to understand and measure risk, and of methods of avoiding them. Several of these are discussed next.

Real Risk Versus Perceived Risk

The fundamental problem that most organizations face in a time of uncertainty is overcoming active imaginations. Without a clear vision of the future, information voids are often filled with wild speculation, manifesting themselves more like worst-case scenarios than realistic assessments of risk. Decision making may be chaotic, yielding the illusion of addressing key issues but using inappropriate tools and analysis.

For instance, assume that a hospital runs "doomsday" scenarios on three independent events: Medicare reimbursement cuts of an additional 20 percent; unionization of 50 percent of the workforce, resulting in a 15 percent increase in salary expense; and losing a managed care contract that accounts for 10 percent of admissions. If each of these events has a 20 percent chance of occurring, the likelihood that all three will happen simultaneously is only 0.8 percent (20 percent times 20 percent times 20 percent). Even though the probability of all three events happening simultaneously is remote, management can sometimes be consumed with the specter of this frightening scenario and overestimate the real risk.

Risk of the Status Quo

A second common pitfall in strategic planning under uncertainty is taking a wait-and-see attitude, hoping facts will reveal themselves in the future and identify the best strategy the organization should undertake. Such an attitude can be the result of multiple, conflicting agendas of decision makers that throw the organization into chaotic gridlock (commonly known as planning paralysis); a false sense of security or complacency (also known as being clueless); a total misreading of the future (referred to as acute myopia); or general lack of leadership.

In the rare case of the status quo being the best strategic alternative, the organization is relying on luck to succeed in the future. Financial planning should include explicit assessment of the risk of maintaining the status quo. For example, what are the risks of not upgrading open-heart surgery facilities? Will this lead to dissatisfaction among patients, physicians, and payers and ultimately to a competitor opening a freestanding heart hospital?

Bracketing the Range of Risk

Knowing that residual uncertainty is present even after the organization's best efforts to identify true risk, additional insight can be gleaned by bracketing the range of projected risk exposure. This is done by estimating the upside and downside risks. Determining how sensitive the financial outcome is to changes in key variables has long been used in financial forecasting to obtain insights that can increase management's comfort with a particular strategic course. This is commonly known as sensitivity analysis and is the financial world's equivalent to scenario planning and decision analysis.

All of these are forms of what-if evaluation tools. For example, if managed care penetration is forecast to increase from 25 percent to 35 percent over the forecast period, a sensitivity analysis testing the impact of a 40 percent penetration can yield insights as to the magnitude of the risk this scenario presents, and determine if such a scenario invalidates the organization's strategic decisions.

A common pitfall when bracketing the risk range is to focus on either end of the bracket. Some organizations allow the excitement of the upside financial reward or fear of the downside financial risk to drive their decisions. A balanced approach is to realize that the specifics of the future are too vague to depend on and that the organization should manage its operations and financial performance within a range that incorporates the best estimates of what can be expected. If performance falls within this range, management assumes that operations are under control; outside the range, corrective actions must be taken.

Risk of Choosing the Wrong Path

A primary concern of decision makers during times of uncertainty is that the likelihood of choosing the wrong strategy is greatly increased. This concern is based on the fact that health care capital is not easily adapted to alternative uses; for example, investment in expanding outpatient services on a hospital's campus cannot be transferred to an off-campus site. Such concerns can lead to gridlock in decision making.

The risk of choosing the wrong path has two major implications for strategic planning. The first is to realize that decisions must be made based on facts available at the time. As the future evolves and new facts surface, the decisions made earlier may no longer be the best available alternatives. If so, then the organization must refocus its efforts, without casting blame for earlier decisions. The lesson is that an organization must maintain a flexible posture with respect to its strategic and financial planning, realizing that it is a dynamic process that requires updating as new facts emerge.

The second implication is that financial capital must be managed prudently. For example, if an organization consumes all of its financial capability implementing a strategy that turns out to be suboptimal, the likelihood of recovery is dramatically reduced. Seldom is such a bet-the-farm strategy warranted. The organization must determine and allocate its financial capability to best ensure the organization's long-term economic viability.

Risk of Throwing Good Money After Bad

No strategy is guaranteed to succeed; therefore, decisions to evaluate divestment versus reinvestment in a "losing" strategy become critical. As discussed in Chapters Five and Seven, organizations should establish and continuously monitor trigger points and metrics, which can serve as important signals for adjusting strategy or quickly identifying and changing a losing one.

Since it may be viewed as admitting failure, many health care organizations are reluctant to confront the difficult decision of divestiture. An extreme example of a decision to back away from a losing strategy was the exit of MedPartners (now Caremark Pharmaceutical Group) from what many saw as its core business, physician practice management. Less extreme examples include provider organizations selling or closing HMOs, which were hot strategies in the mid-1990s. Appropriate and timely divestment, whether it involves selling an operation or ceasing its activity, is often the hallmark of a successful health care company and, as discussed in Chapter Six, is a defining characteristic of a market adapter.

Mitigating Risk

Considering methods to mitigate risks is prudent during periods of uncertainty. Seeking partners to share the risk (another example of market adaptive behavior) and shifting risk are common methods of risk reduction. For instance, several hospitals may partner to establish an HMO, thereby diversifying the risk among several parties. A managed care company may reduce its risk by agreeing to allow capitation payment to providers. Providers accepting capitation may transfer risk by purchasing reinsurance policies. The key factor to evaluate when considering risk reduction strategies is the cost-benefit ratio. For instance, an organization needs to compare the cost of the reinsurance premium against the expected claims.

Classification of Alternative Uses

In our experience, it is helpful to classify potential needs for capital into five major areas:

1. Ensuring ongoing operations
2. Maintaining the core asset base
3. Accumulating financial reserves for contingencies
4. Funding mission activities
5. Financing strategic initiatives

Ensuring Ongoing Operations

Every organization must have funds available to conduct day-to-day business. Historically, it was easy to determine the required level of transactional cash balances through routine cash management techniques such as analyzing daily cash inflows and outflows to determine the minimum cash balance required to ensure prompt payment of bills. However, in uncertain times, cash flows are much less predictable, so a cash cushion must be incorporated into the targeted transactional cash balances. The magnitude of this cushion can be determined by the techniques discussed later in this chapter.

Maintaining the Core Asset Base

It is the fiduciary responsibility of management and the board of a nonprofit organization to maintain the asset base of the organization to meet the health care needs of its community. This requires routine and extraordinary expenditures, in both the short run and the long run. The most common method of identifying amounts to be funded by this pool is through the organization's capital budgeting process.

However, this process can lead to confusion and to arguments as to what constitutes routine capital expenditures versus strategic investments; this is especially true of replacement technology.

A cleaner method is to allocate the full amount of depreciation expense to the maintenance pool, with senior management responsible for allocating monies for routine and nonstrategic maintenance from this pool. But this process opens up the possibility of short-circuiting the strategic investment review process, so limitations must be placed on the types of expenditures considered routine.

Accumulating Financial Reserves for Contingencies

Prudent financial management dictates that an organization maintain financial reserves sufficient to cover the adverse impact of unforeseen events. We call these reserves "safety stock." These safety stock reserves are in addition to working capital funds and other specific-purpose monies. Therefore, safety stock represents only a portion of cash and investment balances. During an era of uncertainty, the funding for and importance of the safety stock increase substantially. Accumulation of a large financial cushion is prudent owing to the increased probability of major unforeseen events during a time of fundamental change in an industry.

There are two general methods for setting safety stock levels. One calculates reserve levels based on debt service levels, the other based upon cash operating requirements. As an example of the former, a national multihospital system targets three years of debt service as its safety stock, under the philosophy that if the system cannot correct the problems causing the decline in profitability within three years, it is facing a major restructuring decision.

As an example of the latter, a medium-sized regional health care system targets 120 days of cash as its safety stock. It has increased this from the prior 60–day target on the basis of the uncertainty caused by managed care penetration in its service area.

From our experience, we would say the latter methodology is more often used. The advantage of this methodology is that it is easily understood; the disadvantage is that it is ad hoc and not based on any sound analysis. This can be particularly problematic in an era of increasing uncertainty. As a third alternative, a reserve may be held that reflects the cost of retrenching the organization, if the selected strategic direction turns out to be wrong, as demonstrated in the next example.

A strategy selected by a health care organization calls for a $30 million investment over a three-year period, with forecast expenditures of $7 million in year one, $15 million in year two, and $8 million in year three. The project is expected to generate $40 million in value over the life of the project, resulting in a net present value of $10 million.

One year into the strategy, it becomes apparent that the value from implementing the strategy will be $20 million, compared to the original forecast of $40 million, on account of shifts in competition, lower payment rates than originally forecast, and lack of physician support. The organization is faced with spending $23 million (that is, the $15 million in year two plus the $8 million in year three) to complete the project but only receiving $20 million in value. The rational decision is to stop investing in this activity and pursue an alternative strategy.

The alternative strategy costs $28 million and is forecast to generate a value of $34 million, a net present value of $6 million in the changed environment. However, to shut down the original strategy, the organization incurs an additional $1 million in retrofitting cost. A safety stock of $6 million would be required to cover this contingency, which includes the difference between the $28 million cost of the alternative strategy and the remaining $23 million committed to the original strategy, plus the $1 million cost to retrofit.

Although this example focuses on a single strategy, it would be appropriate to aggregate the calculated safety stock for the multiple strategic initiatives adopted by the organization. Careful reflection on this case reveals several key requirements in the financial planning process:

- Strategies must be developed for alternative futures, including forecasts of the costs and benefits of each strategy.

- The process is dynamic. Safety stock targets should be modified as the future unfolds.

- Specific rules for tapping into safety stock funds must be established prior to funding the pool. Establishing such rules is discussed later in this chapter.

This process is appropriate for organizations with significant financial capability, but what about organizations with limited resources? Not having funds available for safety stock investments does not mitigate the need for strategic or financial planning. At a minimum, such an organization should have an exit strategy in place in case it cannot maintain financial viability.

Funding Mission Activities

Many health care organizations are driven by a religious mission or have charitable purposes they serve. It is particularly important for these organizations to earmark a portion of their financial capability for these mission purposes. Funding these activities entails unique problems, not the least of which is the argument that "everything we do supports the mission." Consequently, the first step is to define what activities are funded from this "mission" pool. Here is a definition used by a number of organizations; it offers a clear delineation of mission activities:

The activity must be agreed to by the board of directors as advancing the mission or charitable purpose of the organization, prior to approving the expenditures of funds.

The activity is not expected to generate the required risk-adjusted rate of return and will need to be subsidized in some form on an ongoing basis.

Once a mission activity has been identified, its overall cost, including the value of the subsidy, must be calculated. For example, if the activity being considered will cost $2 million in direct costs and is forecast to generate losses of $150,000 per year in perpetuity, the cost of this activity is $3.5 million if the perpetuity is evaluated at 10 percent. Organizations should avoid the temptation of reclassifying to mission activity those activities that turn out to be bad business decisions.

Financing Strategic Initiatives

Strategic initiatives are all investment alternatives that do not fall into the other four categories of investment. During times of great industry change and uncertainty, it is prudent to build a significant war chest, dedicated to strategic initiatives, to allow quick response to changing market conditions.

All strategic initiatives should compete for funding on a common basis, with each alternative ranked by scores using common evaluation criteria. The criteria capture decision-making dimensions unique to the organization and weight them as to relative importance to that organization. Proper design of the evaluation criteria is crucial. They must assign weights to both quantitative and qualitative criteria. For instance, although mission activities rarely produce substantial quantitative returns, their importance is high in nonprofit hospitals. Another example of the quantitative measure alone not reflecting the whole story is the need to invest in new technologies that are required for remaining competitive, some of which can be characterized as loss leaders.

The financial aspects of the criteria should address differing levels of risk by adjusting the required rates of return. For instance, the rate of return for enhancement of a hospital's core business, such as expanding emergency department capacity, would require a significantly lower rate of return than investing in a business in which the hospital has limited expertise, for example, long-term care. Developing and using evaluation criteria is discussed next.

Evaluation Criteria

Applying evaluation criteria to potential capital investments allows rank ordering of alternatives and mitigates much of the politics of investment decision making by ensuring that evaluations are made consistently and objectively. This is not a simple process, especially in health care. It is a complex act to balance the needs of the various constituencies—board members, management, physicians, and the community served—with the organization's ability to meet those needs. Without a structured approach, the decision-making process tends to look ad hoc at best and politically biased at worst. In our experience, using evaluation criteria can help to overcome many of these complexities and facilitate the decision-making process.

There are three major classes of evaluation criteria: mission, financial, and strategic. Mission criteria address the organization's philosophical reasons for existence. Typically, mission-related criteria refer to core purposes such as responding to unmet community needs for services that require subsidy. Financial criteria directly measure the economic impact of a strategic alternative and include such measures as risk-adjusted rate of return, payback period, use of debt, and length of time to breakeven from operations. Strategic criteria capture various aspects of the organization's strategic intent and can include measures of service area expansion, horizontal or vertical integration, and service shifts to less intense settings. The strategic criteria should link to measures of success for the organization, since the latter articulate what the organization is trying to achieve.

There is no single set of criteria applicable to all organizations. Because the players, markets, and missions differ among organizations, sets of criteria are unique to each entity. However, certain general guidelines can be used for developing evaluation criteria:

- Minimize the number of criteria. As with scenario planning, attention should be focused on those with the greatest impact on strategic intent. Again, it is important to link evaluation criteria and measures of success.

- Ensure that the design of each criterion is unambiguous. It is crucial that the intent and measurement of the criteria not be subject to creative interpretation.

- Establish objective and concrete measures for each criterion. For criteria with qualitative measurements, scores should be assigned by a project review committee, not an individual or group championing the initiative.

- Specify the required level of scoring documentation, keeping in mind that a $50,000 alternative does not warrant the same degree of scrutiny as a $50 million alternative. This can serve as the basis for monitoring approved strategic initiatives.

- Recognize that not all criteria are equally important. Scores should reflect the relative importance of each criterion.

Regarding this last point, if for instance the organization's strategic intent is to be a market enactor, then criteria measuring progress in this direction should have higher scores than those met with status quo strategies. Conversely, if an organization has limited financial capability, criteria measuring short-term financial performance should be assigned higher weights than those measuring long-term strategic positioning. In addition, scoring ranges should reflect positive values for "good" forecast outcomes, negative values for "bad" forecast outcomes, and a zero value for forecast outcomes that minimally meet the criterion standards. Using this methodology, alternatives with aggregate negative scores are not acceptable; the remaining alternatives, with aggregate positive scores, are then rank-ordered.

Developing criteria for an organization is an iterative process. They should be identified and discussed, and measurements should be specified by a group, such as the planning committee, that represents the key constituencies of the organization. During the development process, criteria are added and deleted from the initial list and weight assigned to reflect the relative importance of each one. If the process is successful, the resulting set of criteria gives the organization a balanced approach to reviewing strategic initiatives. Table 8.2 contains a sample decision criterion, while Table 8.3 illustrates a sample set of decision criteria.

Quantifying Resource Requirements

Once strategies have been classified into the five types of investment alternatives and evaluation criteria have been developed, the next step is to quantify the resources required to make a strategy

Table 8.2. Sample Evaluation Criteria.

Criterion	Internal rate of return (IRR) compared to risk adjusted discount rate of 12%	
Type	Quantitative	
Scoring	IRR greater than or equal to 14%	10 points
	IRR greater than or equal to 13%, but less 14%	5 points
	IRR greater than or equal to 11%, but less 13%	0 points
	IRR greater than or equal to 10%, but less 11%	−5 points
	IRR less than 10%	−10 points
Scoring responsibility	Finance department	
Rationale	The organization must expect to be compensated for the risk it assumes.	
	Higher returns are preferred to lower returns.	

Table 8.3. Sample Set of Evaluation Criteria.

Criterion	Type	Measurement	Scoring	Responsibility
Collaboration	Quantitative or judgmental	Degree of collaboration with outside partners	• Significant collaboration with new partner (5 points) • Significant collaboration with existing partner (0 points) • No collaboration involved (−5 points)	Evaluation committee with input from planning and managed care departments
Financial risk	Quantitative	Effect of capitation revenue and legislative impacts on cash flow	• Revenue increase > 5% (7 points) • Impact on revenue ≤ 5% (0 points) • Revenue decrease > 5% (−7 points)	Evaluation committee with input from finance and managed care departments
Project breakeven	Quantitative	Number of years until project becomes self-supporting	• < 2 (3 points) • 2–3 (0 points) • > 3 (−5 points)	Evaluation committee with input from finance department
Management expertise	Judgmental	Management expertise available	• In-house expertise available (1 point) • In-house expertise, not easily available (0 points) • No in-house expertise (−1 point)	Evaluation committee with input from administrator of proposing organization
Clinical integration	Judgmental	Level of clinical integration	• Contributes to integration (1 point) • Does not contribute to integration (0 points)	Evaluation committee with input from medical staff and VP of patient care services

happen. There is usually considerable focus on expenditures for the fixed-asset component of the strategy. Equally important, though— and possibly more so—are working capital needs and the human capital required to implement the strategy.

Management often focuses attention on the fixed-asset portion because it is typically the easiest to predict and remains relatively static. However, during times of uncertainty, the focus must shift away from strategies that require long-term commitment in bricks and mortar toward strategies that permit flexibility, that is, to those where the primary investment is working and human capital, which can be more easily shifted. This creates additional challenges for financial planning, since the latter components are more dynamic than equipment or building costs and much more difficult to predict. For example, one possible reason for the financial disappointment of physician acquisition and HMO development strategies was underestimation of the working capital and management resources required to manage both of these activities.

The importance of bracketing the range of acceptable risk and financial performance has already been discussed in this chapter. This task becomes more complex if strategies primarily consume working and human capital because the potential range of outcomes is much wider. In the next sections we offer three techniques that are commonly used to estimate the range of resource requirements. Each successive technique requires a greater degree of financial sophistication than the preceding one. Although they have been used frequently in financial planning, disciplined use of sophisticated techniques takes on great importance during times of uncertainty.

"Guesstimate"

The guesstimate technique uses the judgment of management to come up with the best estimate of the range of outcomes; it should be based on current understanding of the future. For example, if according to historical analysis fifteen days' worth of cash is required for transactions, management may project that at least twice that amount is required to absorb the unknown volatility of the future.

Although better than ignoring the problem, this approach is not recommended.

Sensitivity Analysis

This approach assumes that the organization has a financial plan in place. Still, a financial plan is simply a structured means of examining an organization's future. Because of the many assumptions necessary for financial modeling, even the very best financial plan is unlikely to resolve uncertainty totally or predict the future financial outcome with precision. Therefore, sensitivity analysis is used to bracket the range of risk, as described previously in this chapter.

Recall from Chapter Five that decision analysis and scenario planning are means to evaluate alternative futures. Sensitivity analysis is a variation of these tools, used specifically for financial planning; it imparts structure to quantifying the financial impact of what-if situations. For instance, if a strategic initiative includes redesigning patient care protocols to reduce salary expense, then a sensitivity analysis is run on patient care hours or average direct salaries per patient encounter. This gives some guidance on the range of financial risk of this strategic initiative.

Using an example from Chapter Five, let's assume a hospital is considering purchasing an additional MRI unit and believes that its competitor may follow suit. A series of sensitivity analyses are run on market share and volume. One sensitivity assumes that the hospital purchases the MRI, the competitor does not, the hospital markets the MRI, and the hospital increases market share in MRI services by 20 percent. Another scenario might be that both organizations acquire MRIs, the hospital does not market MRI service, and its MRI market share declines by 10 percent. The results of these two scenarios represent the best and worst financial outcomes of market forces (shown in Figure 5.2). The results of the sensitivity can serve as the basis for determining the cash cushion required and safety stock investments.

Two words of caution are warranted. First, the variables selected for sensitivity analysis should be those uncertainties with the greatest impact on strategic intent. Sensitivity analyses reflecting events with little likelihood of occurring or with limited impact on strategic intent are, at best, a waste of time. At worst they may cause the organization to overfund a strategy, thus diverting resources from activities that can lead to a more viable future.

The second word of caution is not to overinterpret the results of the sensitivity analysis. As previously mentioned, analyzing a doomsday scenario of three independent events each with a 20 percent likelihood of occurrence results in a situation with a 0.8 percent chance of happening. Consequently, summing the adverse impacts of each to determine the cash cushion is equivalent to covering the organization against events that have less than one chance in a hundred of occurring. Even if each event has a 50 percent likelihood, there is only one chance in eight that all three will occur.

This overinterpretation also can occur if residual uncertainty exists and no amount of research yields quantifiable odds of a particular scenario occurring. For example, the future of certificate-of-need (CON) regulations in many states can be viewed as residual uncertainty, as can expansion of Medicare benefits. Each has significant financial implications for health care organizations, and it is essential to quantify the potential impact using sensitivity analysis. However, management should use the results of such financial analyses as a guide rather than a determinant on which to focus substantial attention, since it is impossible to determine the true likelihood of the event(s) happening.

Monte Carlo Simulation: Discussion

Monte Carlo simulation is a statistical technique that addresses the shortcomings of sensitivity analysis by giving appropriate weight to each scenario. Since this is a statistically driven technique, it does require assignment of probabilities to each scenario—a difficult task whenever residual uncertainty exists. Although full discussion of the Monte Carlo technique is beyond the scope of this chapter, a brief discussion and an illustration follow.

Step One: Develop a Model of Variable Behavior

Suppose inpatient demand depends on the use rate of days of inpatient care per thousand population. In management's judgment, there is a 20 percent chance that the use rate will fall in the range of 400–420 days, a 60 percent chance that it will fall between 420 and 450 days, and a 20 percent chance that it will fall between 450 and 470 days.

Step Two: Incorporate the Variable

This can be done on any spreadsheet program.

Step Three: Create Random Scenarios on Variable Distributions

Typically, five hundred to one thousand iterations are run on the variable distributions developed in the first step. The mean and standard deviation then are calculated.

Table 8.4 presents the results of such a simulation for the cash cushion required for a small, newly developed health system. Their baseline scenario indicated that $10.7 million would be needed in 2000, increasing to $11.7 million by 2003. System planners created a simulation model to study the impact of unplanned shifts in Medicare, managed care penetration, and other strategies and interventions that are within the control of the system. Using uniform

Table 8.4. Determination of Cash Cushion (in millions).

	2000	2001	2002	2003
Baseline operating cash	$10.7 m	$11.0 m	$11.4 m	$11.7 m
Simulation results: incremental cash flow:				
Mean	($151,000)	$199,000	$327,000	($402,000)
Standard deviation	$5.6 m	$7.7 m	$9.0 m	$10.4 m
Total cash cushion	$9.0 m	$12.6 m	$14.8 m	$17.2 m

distribution for all parameters, one thousand iterations of the model were performed.

The results summarized in Table 8.4 indicate that the volatility of the cash flows may require another $9.0 million to be held as a cash cushion in 2000, and that this cash cushion requirement can be expected to increase to $17.2 million in 2003, with a 95 percent chance (computed at 1.65 times the standard deviation) that the cash cushion is sufficient to cover downside risks.

A significant challenge in quantifying resource requirements during times of industry restructuring is calculating the collateral and residual impact of each strategy. For instance, a strategy to build a freestanding diagnostic imaging center at the edge of a hospital's primary service area is likely to negatively affect the volume of outpatient radiology procedures performed at the hospital. This is known as a collateral impact and should be included in overall financial evaluation of a strategy. Calculation of a residual impact acknowledges that most strategies are long term and the potential investment or return continues beyond the finite horizon of the financial planning cycle. Therefore, evaluation of the strategy should include some calculation of the residual value of the strategy past the planning horizon under consideration. A perpetuity calculation is the most commonly used method to estimate residual value.

Allocate Resources

Once the organization's financial capability is determined, management must decide how to allocate it to various uses. This entails balancing numerous, conflicting demands for these funds and necessitates certain decisions:

- How will monies be allocated among the operations, safety stock, maintenance, mission, and strategic initiative "buckets," both initially and over time?

- For each allocation, how much of the funding is in the form of cash and how much in unused debt capacity?

- What are the rules for consuming funds from each of
  the five buckets? For instance, what is the maximum
  amount of financial capability that can be consumed in
  each period, and under what conditions is debt issued?

- What events cause the organization to reevaluate its
  allocation process? For example, what if the organization is approached by a hospital willing to sell its
  assets? What if financial performance is considerably
  different from forecasts, resulting in a significant shift
  in the organization's financial capability?

Financial capability is dynamic, reflecting the economic realities that manifest themselves over time. These dynamics also must
be captured in the process. The next example illustrates such a
process.

Allocation of Financial Capability

The "Community Health Corporation" (CHC) has prepared a
financial forecast integrated with its strategic plan; it starts with calculating financial capacity. The forecast sources of financial capability are presented in Table 8.5; allocation of this total financial
capability is discussed next.

Operations Capital

Allocating financial capability to operations has two components:
baseline operating cash and the cash cushion. Allocations for CHC
are summarized in Table 8.6.

Maintenance Capital

CHC's maintenance capital is to be funded annually with an
amount equal to its depreciation expense. Amounts not consumed
during the current year are carried over to the succeeding year. From

Table 8.5. Sources and Uses of Financial Capability (CHC Example) (in millions).

	2000	2001	2002	2003
Sources of financial capability				
Beginning cash and investments	$297.2 m	$318.9 m	$335.8 m	$308.6 m
Annual net cash flows from operations	98.7 m	105.9 m	113.8 m	117.3 m
Fundraising	5.0 m	5.0 m	0	0
Planned borrowing	0	35.0 m	0	0
Available debt capacity	63.2 m	72.0 m	63.7 m	55.0 m
Total sources of financial capability	$464.1 m	$536.8 m	$513.3 m	$480.9 m
Uses of financial capability				
Operations	$19.7 m	$23.6 m	$26.2 m	$28.9 m
Maintenance	50.1 m	101.1 m	80.9 m	58.8 m
Safety stock	127.5 m	128.5 m	130.1 m	133.0 m
Mission	7.0 m	7.0 m	7.0 m	7.0 m
Strategic	259.8 m	276.6 m	269.1 m	253.2 m
Total uses of financial capability	$464.1 m	$536.8 m	$513.3 m	$480.9m

Table 8.6. Allocation of Financial Capability to Operations (CHC Example) (in millions).

	2000	2001	2002	2003
Baseline operating cash	$10.7 m	$11.0 m	$11.4 m	$11.7 m
Cash cushion	9.0 m	12.6 m	14.8 m	17.2 m
Total allocation	$19.7 m	$23.6 m	$26.2 m	$28.9 m

these maintenance amounts, routine replacements and maintenance of the existing facility are funded, ranging from $25.0 million in 2000 to $31.0 million in 2003. A $70.0 million renovation is forecast for 2001 and 2002, half of which is funded with long-term debt. During the forecast period, maintenance capital is funded with $164.8 million from operations and $35.0 million in anticipated borrowing. CHC also has committed $182.0 million in expenditures for short-term and long-term maintenance. By the end of the forecast period, CHC is expected to increase its uncommitted financial capability to $27.8 million. This information is summarized in Table 8.7.

Safety Stock Investment

CHC is targeting sixty days of expenses held in cash to cover strategic contingencies. This methodology was selected instead of others (such as determining the cost of implementing a new strategy) thanks to ease of calculation and the fact that board members are familiar with this measure. In addition, management believes that the amount calculated is sufficient to cover the contingency of having to refocus its strategy. The amount earmarked for safety stock investments is $127.5 million in 2000, increasing to $133.0 million by 2003.

Mission Capital

CHC is mandated to spend an incremental $7 million per year on mission-related activities not already being supported.

Strategic Capital

Financial capability not allocated to operations, maintenance, safety stock, or mission is allocated to strategic capital. As shown in Table 8.8, strategic capital is projected to range from $251.1 million to $276.6 million over the forecast period, with an average annual commitment of $65 million for strategic initiatives. This leaves an uncommitted financial capability, or war chest, of between $173.2 million and $216.6 million during the forecast period each year to invest in new strategic initiatives.

Table 8.7. Allocation of Financial Capability to Maintenance Capital (CHC Example) (in millions).

	2000	2001	2002	2003	Total
Beginning uncommitted financial capability	$10.0 m	$25.1 m	$39.1 m	$16.9 m	$10.0 m
Funding:					
• Depreciation	40.1 m	41.0 m	41.8 m	41.9 m	164.8 m
• Planned borrowing	0	35.0 m	0	0	35.0 m
• Total funding	40.1 m	76.0 m	41.8 m	41.9 m	199.8 m
Total allocated financial capability	50.1 m	101.1 m	80.9 m	58.8 m	209.8 m
Committed uses of capital					
• Routine maintenance	25.0 m	27.0 m	29.0 m	31.0 m	112.0 m
• Renovation	0	35.0 m	35.0 m	0	70.0 m
• Total uses	25.0 m	62.0 m	64.0 m	31.0 m	182.0 m
Ending uncommitted financial capability	$25.1 m	$39.1 m	$16.9 m	$27.8 m	$27.8 m

Table 8.8. Allocation of Financial Capability to Strategic Capital (CHC Example) (in millions).

	2000	2001	2002	2003
Allocated financial capability				
• Cash	$196.6 m	$204.6 m	$205.4 m	$198.2 m
• Available debt capacity	63.2 m	72.0 m	63.7 m	55.0 m
• Total	259.8 m	276.6 m	269.1 m	253.2 m
Committed uses of capital	50.0 m	60.0 m	70.0 m	80.0 m
Uncommitted financial capability	$209.8 m	$216.6 m	$199.1 m	$173.2 m

CHC management has as a target that no more than 25 percent of the uncommitted financial capability be consumed in any one year for projects generated through the budgeting process. Further, all projects and strategies compete for funding on an equal basis using a standard evaluation process; they are then ranked by scores received from applying CHC evaluation criteria. Once an investment alternative is approved, an amount equal to the funding requirement is reclassified from the uncommitted to the committed strategic capital financial capability.

Other than prudent financial management, limiting the annual commitment to no more than 25 percent of uncommitted strategic capital financial capability also gives CHC the flexibility to respond to new strategic alternatives that reveal themselves after the budgeting process. Further, it can serve as an additional buffer to any adverse turn of events whose financial impact cannot be completely absorbed by the cash cushion.

Reexamining Financial Capability

Since financial capability is dynamic, its calculation and allocation must be reexamined periodically, at least annually, as part of the budgeting process or whenever significant events affect the organization. For example, if managed care penetration and discounts are significantly greater than originally projected, the organization's strategic focus must be reexamined to determine if the current direction is valid or if financial capability should be recalculated. Assuming in our previous example that annual cash flows are forecast to decrease by 50 percent, not only are available investment balances reduced by $218 million but the ability to borrow funds is eliminated. The total impact on financial capability is $272 million. If, as a result of the decreased cash flows, CHC is unable to borrow the $35 million in 2001, its available investment balances would be reduced by $253 million and its financial capability reduced by $307 million by 2003.

There are six key issues to resolve in reexamining financial capability:

1. Should the cash cushion be applied to reduced financial capability?

2. Should the organization revisit its commitment to maintenance capital?

3. Are these events of the type that triggers use of safety stock investments?

4. Can mission capital be maintained at targeted levels?

5. Should strategic capital commitments be reevaluated?

6. How have these events affected the ability to attract lenders, and what impact does this have on risk tolerance? For instance, is CHC willing to position itself as a riskier borrower by accepting more restrictive loan terms such as higher borrowing rates and contractual limitations on investment activities?

The first five questions in the list focus on shifting dollars from the representative buckets to the strategic capital pool. Question six has an impact on the organization's incremental debt capacity.

There are no hard-and-fast rules on how funding priorities should be shifted in light of such a significant impact on financial capability. Each organization has to decide on its own, from the best information available. For less dramatic shifts, the focus of the impact is ordinarily on reallocating strategic capital.

Conclusion

Financial planning reflects the realities of today's health care environment: limited resources, seemingly limitless options, and no clear direction in the health care environment. Financial planning is a complementary structure to strategic decision making. Integrating financial and strategic planning has always been important, but it takes on critical importance during times of uncertainty while financial resources are dwindling.

An objective and disciplined process of allocating financial resources requires mechanisms to incorporate risk assessment systematically into financial evaluation of alternative strategic initiatives. A strong financial planning process can mitigate some of the risks of uncertainty and help ensure future success and continued viability. Financial planning and modeling require making assumptions about the future. Therefore, a financial plan is only as good as the assumptions and characteristics built into it. However, even the best model should not supplant sound management judgment.

Lessons Learned

✓ Financial planning is a balancing act that occurs at the highest levels of the organization, matching the financial demands associated with strategic intent with the supply of capital resources. However, it also occurs on lower levels in the form of balancing the risk of uncertainty with the reward of success, and balancing capital among various types of need.

✓ Successful financial planning depends on objectively identifying and weighing risks and using a disciplined approach to allocating resources.

✓ Debt capacity is dynamic; each strategic decision has an impact on the funds available for other strategic initiatives.

✓ Financial capability can be volatile in uncertain times and must be reevaluated, at least annually, to form the foundation of refining or revising strategic intent.

✓ It is prudent to build a war chest to allow the organization to respond quickly to the unpredictable future of the health care industry.

✓ During times of uncertainty, the focus shifts away from strategies that require long-term commitment in bricks and mortar toward strategies that rely on working and human capital, which can be more easily shifted than investments in buildings.

Ensuring Success in Implementation

Marian C. Jennings and J. Edward Witek

Strategic intent has value only if it can be implemented success-fully. What is it that allows one organization to commit to and smoothly implement its plan, while another continues to endlessly debate or revisit key components? How can your organization learn from past mistakes and move on, not letting past failures haunt current efforts? What is the right balance between a consensus-driven approach and a leadership-driven one? What approaches to enlist stakeholders as change agents work best?

This chapter explores the difficulties in implementing strategic intent in an increasingly uncertain environment, and the linkages between strategic intent and organizational style. Critical factors are identified that enhance success during plan implementation, as well as practical approaches for managing the human side of change. The chapter concludes with a discussion of how measures of success can be used to keep implementation efforts on track.

Escaping the Graveyard of Failed Change Efforts

Traditionally, strategy implementation has required well-defined tactics, clear-cut responsibilities and authorities, and articulation of challenging but achievable time frames. Even in a stable environment, successful implementation was difficult and created competitive advantages for those organizations that mastered it. Successful health care organizations often have a long history of successfully implementing their previous vision(s) and goals, with decades of favorable results.

Today, many of these same organizations are reeling from their lack of success or outright failures in implementing recent strategic initiatives, such as attempts to diversify, to excel at niche specialization, to attach "covered lives" to their system, to become the Nordstrom's of health care service quality, or to integrate along the continuum of care. These unexpected failures, often of bold big-bet strategies, have reinforced the generally risk-averse culture of the industry. Board members, senior and midlevel managers, physician leaders, and staff alike have become desensitized by a steady stream of proposed "strategic visions." In a vision-fatigued environment, managers and staff often lack the drive to take risks; instead they opt for measured steps to show support until an initiative is abandoned. Each failed strategy adds to hesitation to make significant and timely change.

As an example, a regional health care system recently promoted its chief operating officer to the CEO slot and used the opportunity to reexamine its strategic plan. The existing plan, crafted in the mid-1990s largely by the former CEO, boldly called for strategic repositioning of the organization as a fully integrated delivery and financing system. The plan's targets included doubling market share, expanding its geographic market, rapidly acquiring primary care physician practices, joint venturing with an insurer to introduce a branded managed care product, and focusing on three clinical centers of excellence. The system developed detailed implementation plans with well-defined tactics, clear-cut responsibilities and authorities, and expected timetables. Competent, experienced managers devoted significant time and resources to implement the plan.

Despite its well-articulated strategy, the system has failed to achieve most if not all of its strategic objectives, experiencing market share declines and financial performance that continued spiraling downward. Primary care and specialist physicians saw the primary care physician strategy as unfocused. The joint-ventured insurance product failed to materialize since no area insurers were interested in developing a provider-branded product, and consumers could not differentiate the system's centers of excellence from those of its competitors. Physicians, who had never supported much of the original plan or the former CEO (whom they viewed as autocratic), were very happy to participate in a new "reality-based" planning process.

The results of the process? The organization could reach consensus only on the need to enhance its financial performance and rebuild physician-system relationships. Although leaders articulated their desire for the system to be a flexible market adapter, the initiatives they endorsed were those of a market survivor. They were a battle-weary group. Six months later, no specific actions other than continued cost reduction had been identified to improve financial performance, and no specific approaches formulated to enhancing relationships with physicians. Most of the momentum that accompanied a change in CEO leadership had dissipated. Trying to reenergize the planning group, especially its physician members, and restore credibility to the planning process were now challenging tasks.

What could have been done differently in this organization, and in numerous similar situations?

First, recognize that successful planning and implementation in an era of uncertainty require a directive senior leadership role. The CEO must be seen as personally committed to a successful planning effort. He or she must push the organization to achieve its fullest strategic potential. In our example, the new CEO was so hesitant about being seen as autocratic that he relinquished his leadership role and agreed to pursue weak, vague goals that felt comfortable to the group.

Second, openly acknowledge the reality of uncertainty and its impact on the organization's ability to ensure successful implementation. Especially in organizations used to success, the tendency is to ignore or rationalize past strategic failures or to attribute the failure to a departed individual. No one wants to admit that today's strategic plan also may fail to achieve its objectives. This is an example of the "elephant in the room" phenomenon; fear of failure virtually immobilizes the organization, but no one talks about the fear. Instead, as in our example, no-regrets-move strategies dominate the strategic intent under the mistaken belief that, since such initiatives are more under the organization's control, they are a less risky overall strategy.

Successful organizations take decisive action despite uncertainty. To mitigate the immobilizing fear of failure, planning participants as a group should review the assumptions that drove the organization's strategies in the past, openly discuss what has changed, identify what went well or poorly in prior implementation efforts, and agree to use this learning to help the organization increase its chances of future success. Participants must accept that no one can guarantee future success.

Third, help participants to understand and endorse two practical ways to reduce the risks of large-scale, visible failure in implementation. The first is to use well-defined feedback mechanisms, such as the measures of success discussed in Chapter Seven, in shortened periods of, say, six-month intervals. The second is to purposely be flexible in changing strategies and tactics, when needed, to achieve desired results.

Last of all, work with leaders at all levels to accept that strategic planning in an era of uncertainty often requires transformational change, not incremental change. Such change may appear to be an assault on the foundations of the organization. To mitigate this concern, make sure that the planning process is founded on a clear, compelling core ideology, as outlined in Chapter Six.

In addition, a hazard to all organizations undertaking transformational change is overlooking or minimizing the human side of change. Change is often unsettling at both the personal and professional levels. For example, health care executives working through a merger or acquisition are regularly dismayed to find that the process has taken years, not months. Relationships, feedback, and traditional measures for evaluating success all may be changed. Management must clearly and regularly communicate a consistent message regarding the long-term vision and progress toward that vision. In the absence of information, perceptions about expectations and timing can become dominated by rumor and gossip. Without constant communication and consistent reassurance, dysfunctional behaviors grow, including risk aversion, passive aggressiveness, self-protective actions, or the departure of key contributors.

Matching Strategic Intent and Organizational Style

Implementing strategic intent requires a match between the strategic intent and the organization's culture. In our experience, in a clash between strategic intent and culture, the latter prevails. For example, if a conservative, risk-averse organization selects a market-enactor intent, as described in Chapter Six, a year later it is likely that the board and senior management will still be debating the assumptions underlying the plan. No major market moves will occur since the organization cannot be persuaded that the chances of visible failure are tolerably low.

Although many years old now, the framework of Raymond Miles and Charles Snow (1978) is still an immensely valuable tool for understanding organizational styles. This classic framework (Table 9.1) identified four prototype organizational styles: prospectors, analyzers, defenders, and reactors. Miles and Snow believed that organizations with any of the first three styles could succeed, but the reactor ultimately would fail.

Prospectors

Prospector organizations embrace change. They see change as creating opportunities for their organization, and they often serve as change agents themselves. This style directly matches the strategic

Table 9.1. Organizational Style and Strategic Intent.

Organizational Style	Strategic Intent	Cultural Style	Organizational Structure	Vulnerabilities	Examples
Prospector	Promotes innovation and redefines competitive environment Difficult for competitors to anticipate prospectors' next moves Seeks to develop new products or services to exploit new opportunities in a dynamic environment	Risk taking rewarded Highly collaborative within workgroups	Autonomous workgroups or product divisions Planning and control are highly decentralized	Being able to identify and make the right bets Become overly reliant on a single technology Poaching of key talent by competitors	Oxford Health Plan Columbia/HCA (circa 1997) Humana
Analyzer	Fast follower to prospectors Analysis and imitation Seeks to internalize design and production of new innovation and produce it more cheaply and faster than prospector	Seeks systematic, incremental change	Matrix structure, seeking benefits of both functional and product- or service-oriented organizations	Attack from niche players Low-cost producers	Many Catholic hospitals and systems Many "top 100" hospitals

Defender	Searches for market stability Targets narrow market with a limited product line Has dominant position, which it seeks to defend through barriers to entry Tends to compete on cost or value	Values stability Rewards implementers and cost-cutters	Functional organization Centralized decision making and control Vertical communications and integration High degree of technical specialization	Large shifts in the environment, e.g., keyhole surgery's impact on cardio-vascular surgery	Academic medical centers
Reactor	Does not anticipate market changes or develop strategies to cope with them Reacts to the market Constrained by limited or misallocated resources	No defined organizational style; depends on the circumstances	Organizational structure is misaligned with the needs of the environment and the internal culture	Any particular state of the environment could pose a threat: stability, dramatic change, or incremental change	Isolated community hospital in a rural setting

Source: Adapted from Miles and Snow (1978).

intent of the market enactor. A classic example of a prospector style in health care is Humana, an organization that has transformed itself numerous times over its history. Starting out as a nursing home chain, it became a hospital chain, introduced the concept of urgent care centers, entered the managed care business, and finally divested its core hospital business and attached its strong brand name to an insurance product. In our experience, most examples of market-enactor organizations exhibiting the prospector organizational style occur in the for-profit health care sector.

Analyzers

Analyzer organizations use thorough analysis and careful, systematic processes to reduce their strategic risks. They are rarely the first in a region to implement a strategy, but as quick followers they often implement the refined strategy better than others. This style matches most closely the strategic intent of the market adapter. Most successful not-for-profit health care organizations demonstrate the analyzer style. As appropriate in organizations that are stewards of the community's resources, they are not comfortable pioneering untested, potentially risky strategies without having performed extensive analyses.

In periods of great uncertainty, organizations characterized by the analyzer style can find it difficult to be as flexible and adaptive as required of true market adapters. Their desire to analyze similar situations may be thwarted when industry twins are difficult to identify. They may find their energy for a strategy sapped by the desire to analyze away all risks. This can cause implementation efforts that began with gusto to run out of creativity and energy.

Defenders

Defender organizations seek to maintain the current power structure in the industry and within their own organizations. Defender styles are exhibited most commonly in historically successful and powerful organizations, those articulating the adage "If it ain't broke, why fix it?" The strong culture and commonly held values that typically permeate defender cultures, including a mythology reinforced through years of success, would normally be a great strength. However, under uncertain conditions, holding on to values may manifest itself as a stubborn commitment to what used to work (as in "It's what got us here today"). Finally, defender cultures are particularly susceptible to a related problem called active inertia (Sull, 1999). In this version of inertia, action-oriented managers respond with a flurry of the old, familiar approaches but do not seek new solutions.

Many academic medical centers (AMCs) demonstrate the defender style. For example, AMCs currently are fighting to maintain funding for teaching as an integral component of payment rates and to restore the funding formula to historical levels. Alternative approaches that could conceivably yield as many dollars or more and reward truly outstanding teaching programs are rarely discussed.

The defender style matches most closely the market-survivor strategic intent. That is, the defender often focuses on internal issues and changes incrementally, not radically.

Reactors

Reactor organizations have no consistent approach to the market. They tend always to react to market trends, even reversing course. Reactors survive in today's health care environment only because they operate in isolated markets with little or no competition or managed care pressure, or because they hold substantial endowments. Many of these organizations have already merged (or soon will) into proactive systems.

As leadership changes, organizations can and often do change their organizational style. Columbia/HCA demonstrated an aggressive market-enactor intent built upon an entrepreneurial, prospector style in assembling its portfolio of hospitals, surgery centers, home health, and other concerns nationwide. In Ohio, for example, Columbia/HCA challenged the status quo in its (ultimately unsuccessful) efforts to purchase Blue Cross. With the departure of its aggressive founder, Columbia/HCA has turned into a market survivor characterized by an analyzer style, focusing on reducing costs and disassembling its health care portfolio.

Involving Key Stakeholders in Strategic Formulation and Implementation

Health care organizations have been described for decades as three-legged stools, reflecting the unique and complex interrelatedness of the three major constituency groups of the organization: the board, senior management, and physician leaders. In a slowly changing health care environment, consensus-driven strategic planning and decision making thrived. Achieving consensus before acting was the safest route to ensuring that the plan would be implemented.

The term *consensus* means general agreement. Unfortunately, in too many organizations, the term consensus has come to mean universal agreement or unanimity. Selected individuals, most notably physician leaders or isolated board members, often believe that the organization cannot or should not move forward until every member of the group fully supports the decision. This notion of consensus can be fatal to an organization operating in an environment as dynamic and uncertain as health care. It gives individuals implicit veto power over strategic direction. No organization in a dynamic environment would agree that the pace of change should be dictated by the person least willing to change.

An example of the dangers of expecting universal consensus in strategy formulation emerges from studying the formation of physician-hospital organizations. Many PHOs were formed without working through the difficult relationship and partnership issues among the physicians themselves. Many of the policy decisions related to forming the PHO, including physician credentialing, creating physician panels, and physicians' being willing to participate in single-signature contracting were decided by universal consensus, which de facto became a lowest-common-denominator approach—that is, decisions that would not offend any participant. Consensus-driven organizations were still congratulating themselves about their inclusive process in PHO formation even as they discovered that their new PHOs would not run.

Strategy formulation in an era of uncertainty needs to increase, not reduce, the number of channels for formal input to the process, and to engage key stakeholders in articulating the strategic direction. However, participants need to understand clearly that input is not the same as decision-making responsibility. It is incumbent upon the organization's leaders to weigh the situation, take into account the input of key constituency groups, and then make the difficult decisions, even when selected constituencies are fearful of the outcome or might prefer a less controversial path.

Implementing Strategic Intent: Critical Success Factors

The exhilaration of defining a new strategic intent can quickly turn into organizational frustration. Sadly, many attempts to enact profound change die in the early phases of implementation owing to lack of shared vision or insufficient urgency. As shown in Table 9.2, four critical success factors early in the process can help management establish and sustain momentum in the planning process. Five additional success factors focus on defining and supporting new roles and responsibilities during implementation. Throughout the implementation of strategic intent, the organization must remain flexible, constantly monitoring and adapting on the basis of its performance against measures of success. Finally, there must be continuing awareness of the fit between the strategic intent and the changing environment.

Establish a Broad-Based Sense of Urgency for Change

As the organization's strategic intent is announced, a compelling case must be made supporting the need for change. During the planning process, direct participants come to understand the need for

Table 9.2. Critical Success Factors.

Success Factor	Communication	Desired Result
Early Factors		
Create a sense of urgency	Status quo not viable Action required	Overcome inertia Energize organization
Create a powerful core of supporters	Change has support Rewards outweigh risks	Build momentum with champions; sway doubters
Address concerns of detractors	Opposing opinions are valued Contingency plans are in place	Constructive discussions Gain insight about obstacles
Communicate the vision	Visualization of organization after change Benefits of change	Enhance willing-ness to change Establish common goals
During Implementation		
Establish clear roles and responsibilities	Performance expectations Training, coaching, support structures are available	Understanding of role and objectives Organizational learning
Anticipate manage-ment and staff fallout	Not everyone can thrive in new organization Everyone treated fairly and with respect	Support and learning opportunities provided New leaders step forward; good people retained
Plan and celebrate short-term wins	Progress being made End result worth the effort	Maintain momentum with tangible results Refocus and energize
Institutionalize the changes	New organization is here to stay (incentives, rewards structure)	Change embodied in leaders, policies, and attitudes
Systematize organizational learning	Continuous learning is vital to success	Effective feedback used to modify strategies and tactics in a timely manner

change as well as the alternatives considered and their associated risks. But what about the rest of the organization?

Leaders are often surprised when the broader group of constituents does not share the planning committee's insight and sense of urgency. Senior management, led by the CEO, must communicate a succinct message to physicians, managers, staff, and the community-at-large about the need for change. The message, presented almost endlessly to small groups and one-on-one, must contain an uncomplicated description of what the organization will look like with the realization of strategic intent, and what it will look like if it simply continues on the same path.

Create a Powerful Core of Supporters

Many constituents throughout the organization may not initially appreciate the new strategic intent. Others will question it as they begin to feel the discomfort caused by early change. Senior management, united behind the defined strategic intent, must explain, lobby, cajole, and otherwise secure the support of key leaders on the board and among the medical staff.

Creating supporters occurs through disclosure of organizational needs and alternatives. One-on-one meetings with each potential supporter often are needed to discuss the potential risks and rewards of alternatives for the organization and for them personally. Contingency plans for the riskiest strategies being pursued should be developed and shared with potential key supporters. Such plans can build their confidence in and willingness to support the strategic intent.

Address Concerns of Plan Detractors

There should be a proactive, continuous approach to addressing the objections of those who are not likely to agree with the strategic intent or the need for change, especially transformational change. By including potential objectors in the planning process in clearly defined roles, management takes a calculated risk that one or more positive outcomes will occur—specifically, that:

- Discussions outside the meetings, stimulated by the process, will result in greater understanding

- The opportunity to air views during the process may diminish or delay active opposition to the plan

- The objector may have insight concerning potential risks or obstacles, which facilitates development of contingency plans and effective implementation steps

Potential objectors can be incorporated into the strategy development process in several ways. One or two such individuals can be added to the planning committee, giving them an official forum for articulating their views throughout the process. In this case, it is critical that they understand that no one—themselves included— holds a veto power over the committee's recommendations. Alternatively, potential objectors can participate through confidential one-on-one interviews or on task forces convened to address specific issues.

Communicate the Strategic Intent and Vision Early and Often

An early turning point in the process is communicating the strategic intent and vision outside of the planning group. To sustain the momentum of the planning process, the vision must be communicated frequently, clearly, and concisely. Descriptions of the vision should include what the organization will look like once strategic intent is realized; the benefits of the change to patients, the community, the medical staff and the staff and associates; and expected competitive or sustainable advantage resulting from the strategic plan.

Presentation of the new strategic intent should demonstrate commitment from the board, management, and physician leaders, and include actions and symbols consistent with the new direction. Especially if the organization has been through many new strategic visions before, potential supporters will be listening critically for specific details of the plan. Of great interest will be announcements of timetables, specific management or organizational changes, or planned capital expenditures. For example, an announcement concerning the composition of the implementation planning team and its charge is more credible than vague promises about limiting staff reductions.

Establish Clear Roles, Responsibilities, and Relationships for Implementation

The first of the five factors critical to successful implementation is to establish clear roles for all parties.

If the best way to learn is by doing, then implementing strategic intent generates a bonanza of personal and professional growth opportunities. Transformational change requires managers to work across established organizational and reporting boundaries to restructure or reconfigure services. Each manager, whether leading or participating in the implementation process, should be given the opportunity, direction, resources, and delegated authority to succeed. New definitions of authority, reporting relationships, expectations, incentives, and feedback mechanisms often are required.

Implementation of strategic intent must be managed actively, including clear definition of roles and expectations. Beyond the thoughtfully constructed implementation plan, many organizations have found using a transition team or task forces to be a successful approach. Transition team or task force participants typically include appropriate senior management representatives, various line managers, physicians, and clinicians. The team or task force focuses on accomplishing specific implementation objectives by meeting regularly to report on progress, to discuss and resolve difficult issues, to redefine or reset goals or time frames, or to recommend new action steps. A representative of senior management typically is charged with sustaining the energy and focus of the transition team or task force.

Anticipate Management and Staff Fallout

Some managers and staff cannot adapt to their new roles and responsibilities, particularly in an organization trying to migrate from a reactor or defender style to an analyzer style. It is not uncommon for organizations undergoing transformational change to lose half or more of their management staff. However, an experienced group of managers that already knows how to work together as an effective team can be a strategic asset to an organization undergoing major internal changes in a turbulent marketplace. Senior management should work hard to identify and support those managers who they feel have the potential to grow and learn through their experiences.

A critical question in this phase of implementation concerns when to determine that a manager does not possess the skills and core competencies needed by the organization in the future. Changing managers too early in the implementation process may damage morale and undercut authority. Waiting until a manager has failed can damage both the individual and the organization. It is often beneficial to use an objective third party, skilled in assessing the core competencies, values, and motivations of members of the management team, prior to implementing major transformational change efforts.

Plan for and Celebrate Short-Term Wins

The challenge of sustaining organizational energy and drive can overwhelm and stall implementation before strategic intent is fully realized. By its nature, transformational change takes a heavy toll on everyone in the organization. During the transition period, managers and staff create new systems and learn new ways of working together. Interim lower productivity levels may create frustration and engender feelings of incompetence or lowered self-esteem. As time continues to pass without seeing any of the promised benefits, doubts may begin to fester and critics may grow louder and bolder (Bridges, 1991).

One way to mitigate the doubts and frustrations is to plan for and ensure successes during the transition period. Short-term wins build confidence. Successes may be targeted for pilot programs in a restricted geographic area or in a single service line. Such smaller efforts are easier to control and permit refinement of assumptions and action steps. "Quick successes reassure believers, convince the doubters, and confound the critics" (Bridges, 1991, p. 62).

Finally, take the time to celebrate the small wins by recognizing the team that contributed to the success. The celebrations should reinforce how these small efforts dovetail with the organization's overall vision and strategic intent.

Institutionalize the Changes

As managers, physicians, and staff learn new ways of working, the organizational memory is born anew. With consistent rewards to the change leaders, organizational attitudes are better prepared and confidence is gained for the next transformation. The benefits are ingrained in the organization as the process of identification and development of the next generation of change agents continues.

Systematize Organizational Learning

Health care organizations must develop structured organizational learning mechanisms if they are to capture hard-won lessons and build on both their mistakes and successes. Learning organizations are able to continuously update and revise their strategies to incorporate collective learning. There are three common mechanisms that help to develop a learning organization: the transition team or task force approach (previously discussed), double-loop learning, and the after-action review.

Double-loop learning is the process of capturing both the top-down learning generated during the strategic planning process and the bottom-up learning initiated at the line manager and staff levels (Kaplan and Norton, 1996a). By systematically gathering and analyzing bottom-up lessons learned, organizations can better adapt to unanticipated opportunities and changes in the market.

In his book *Hope Is Not a Method* (1996), former U.S. Army Chief of Staff Gordon R. Sullivan describes the mechanism that the army used to develop itself into a learning organization. Many businesses have since adopted the army's approach, known as the after-action review (AAR). The AAR is a tool to capture organizational lessons learned immediately after every major operational event. The goal of the AAR is to have the leaders involved in the event sit down together and answer the basic questions: What happened? Why did it happen? What should be done about it?

The AAR is more than just a critique of success or failure; it is a tool to capture the lessons to be learned from the organizational experience. To be most effective, the AAR should be developed as a routine event at all levels to systematically build an organizational base of knowledge. Health care organizations typically have in place a clinical version of AAR, often called the "mortality and morbidity conference," which meets to review and learn from patients whose cases were complex or took an unexpected turn.

Adapting the Organization to Risk Taking

As discussed earlier in this chapter in the overview of organizational styles, few not-for-profit health care organizations consistently demonstrate a prospector style. Instead, most community-based or religious-sponsored organizations demonstrate a culture that ranges from somewhat to very risk-averse. What can be done to increase the risk tolerance in your organization's culture?

In the corporate world, U.S. industries transformed themselves over the course of a decade or so to compete effectively in the global markets. Their focus was on changing from a bureaucratic culture to one characterized by prudent risk taking. These organizations focused on five actions that can serve health care organizations equally well today (see Figure 9.1):

1. Reduce the number of management layers for approval. Eliminating opportunities for managers to reject change promotes adoption of initiatives.

2. Demonstrate flexibility, recognizing that implementation cannot always be a linear process; instead it requires quick responsiveness to unforeseen market opportunities or threats.

3. Openly communicate and encourage positive public discussion of failed innovations and initiatives as part of the learning process. As Henry Ford said, "One who fears failure limits his activities. Failure is only the opportunity more intelligently to begin again" (Goodman, 1997, p. 269).

4. Reward risk takers by recognizing and rewarding them even if their efforts are not immediately or completely successful. By doing so, the message becomes ingrained that innovation is expected from all members of the organization.

5. Commit financial resources to support risk-taking endeavors by managers.

Senior Management's Role

Senior management must visibly lead the implementation of strategic intent. This leadership role, which cannot be delegated, is focused and comprehensive, specific and figurative. The CEO and management team must energize, explain, lead by example, listen sympathetically, and still take decisive action. Senior management also should lead celebrations of successes.

Figure 9.1. Five Actions to Create a Risk-Taking Organization.

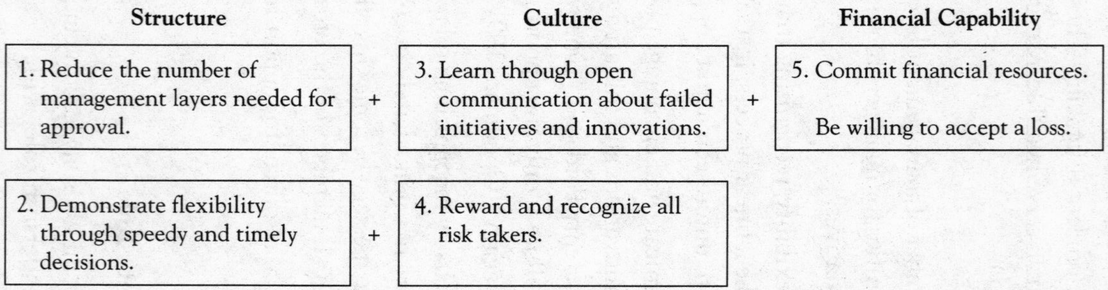

Structure		Culture		Financial Capability
1. Reduce the number of management layers needed for approval.	+	3. Learn through open communication about failed initiatives and innovations.	+	5. Commit financial resources. Be willing to accept a loss.
2. Demonstrate flexibility through speedy and timely decisions.	+	4. Reward and recognize all risk takers.	+	

Senior management must accurately estimate resistance to change and lack of immediate understanding of and support for the strategic intent. Constant communications to groups and in one-on-one sessions should explain strategic intent and keep the organization informed about progress and setbacks.

Senior management must define expectations, align organizational structures, and coach the people who implement the change. Leaders select and enforce measures of success, create incentives for change, and ultimately determine whether the implementation process is working.

Senior management's leadership role is perhaps greatest in managing the human side of change. The transition period—the time between the end of the old ways and establishment of strategic intent—can be an emotional time for many. Wise managers consider these suggestions before acting during the transition:

- Provide accurate information. Do not promise what you cannot deliver (such as job security), and truthfully share information on successes and failures.

- Acknowledge losses openly, with sympathy. Know who will be affected (such as those implementing a new information system) or who will be transferred or terminated.

- Expect and accept signs of grieving. Loyalty to how things have been done often has been imbedded and reinforced by the culture. Do not confuse grieving with poor morale.

- Compensate for losses where you can. Identify what is being lost that is valuable, including status, team membership, or recognition, and offer some appropriate compensation such as training, visibility, or a dignified exit.

- Treat the past with respect. Mark the end of the era by honoring past efforts and accomplishments, while reinforcing the value of the future direction (Bridges, 1991).

The Board's Role

Board members have a fiduciary responsibility for the viability and vitality of the organization. In the early phases of implementation, the board may be exposed to more of the tumult and chaos of change than to any successes and tangible results. The board's informed commitment to the organization's vision and strategic intent is imperative. Informed commitment means that from the beginning and throughout implementation, the board must fully understand the potential capital and human costs of change, accept the risks associated with strategic intent, and be prepared to allocate or reallocate the resources needed to achieve the agreed-upon objectives.

To accomplish its role, the board must:

- Be well educated about the health care industry and the local health care market, including community needs and environmental and competitive trends; have a realistic assessment of organizational positioning and capabilities; and understand the risk and uncertainty implicit in the environment.

- Have in place a governance structure that facilitates effective and efficient decision making.

- Identify and use core competencies and formal qualifications for nominating and appointing board members. All too often, board seats are filled with individuals based solely on relationships, not incorporating the skill sets and abilities needed to ensure that the board can perform its oversight role credibly. Selection criteria also should include willingness and ability to devote the time needed for ongoing education.

- Demand and receive sufficient feedback during plan implementation. How many boards understood the risk of provider-sponsored HMOs until the losses began to mount? Feedback and progress reports are essential to the board's role in safeguarding the organization's resources.

Physician Leaders' Role

Physician leaders must be partners in the change process, acting as change agents with their colleagues and employees (especially their nursing colleagues) to implement strategic intent. Physicians should participate visibly in planning and implementation so that physician leaders can stand alongside management throughout the process of announcing and explaining strategic intent, action steps, implementation successes and failures, and rewards and recognition.

Physician leaders can be valuable assets in assessing future uncertainties, as discussed in Chapters Four and Five, particularly around risks associated with clinical technology advances and with likely reactions from the physician community to a particular initiative. Physician "champions" must be identified during the planning process and actively involved in implementation planning.

Role of Divisional or Departmental Directors

Implementation of the plan at the divisional or department level often proves to be the most difficult step in the process. Senior management must ensure "task alignment" of roles and responsibilities of divisional leaders with strategic intent. Task alignment means focusing energy on overcoming obstacles to change, not on abstractions such as symbolic participation or culture. In pursuing implementation of the change process, division and departmental leaders should rely on three principles:

1. *Communication.* Midlevel managers must be able to articulate the organizational vision and strategic intent, thereby energizing employees to modify tasks and behaviors as needed.

2. *Action plan development.* Managers must be able to develop and implement detailed action plans with achievable timetables, using identified organizational assets.

3. *Organizational capability.* Managers must be empowered to identify and arrange for the additional training or other resources that are required to achieve transformational change.

Managers must maintain focus on organizational goals specific to their divisions. They also can engender broad organizational support throughout the implementation process by working across functional and structural divisions. However, each divisional manager, collaborating with his or her transition team and senior management, must work for successful implementation of strategic intent using three key criteria:

1. Measurement of the impact of change efforts, including ensuring collection of valid and reliable feedback on measurements of success.

2. Alignment of the division and department goals with overall organization goals and strategies.

3. Creation and continuing modification of action steps that yield a positive impact on implementation.

Using a Strategic Feedback System

As described in Chapter Seven, effective feedback systems are always important in implementing strategic intent, but especially so in periods of uncertainty. Planning under uncertainty requires greater responsiveness to the environment and more flexibility in altering actions to achieve the targeted impact. Not all action steps will be known at the time the vision is announced. Measures of success aid in identifying needed changes to actions, strategies, and goals, or even to the strategic intent itself.

Kaplan and Norton (1996a) identify five mechanisms that organizations can use to develop feedback systems to test the effectiveness of their strategic plans: correlation analysis, management gaming, anecdotal reporting, initiative review, and peer review. Each of these is relevant to health care organizations implementing strategic intent.

Correlation Analysis

Health care managers should expect to see a correlation among various performance measures during implementation. By anticipating and measuring the relationship between performance measures, managers can better judge the effectiveness of their selected strategies. For example, one regional system assumed that expanding its primary care referral base in a targeted market would correlate with increased share in that market. The system expanded its primary care base in a market by over 20 percent but realized no market share growth. This might indicate an oversupply of primary care physicians in the area, or high-profile specialists associated with a competitor continuing to pull referrals thanks to the strength of their reputations. The conclusion: the primary care growth strategy is not the expected performance driver for the strategic objective of enhancing market share. This type of feedback enables the organization to better determine what the actual performance driver should be for strategic objectives and initiatives.

Management Gaming

Gaming is an exercise in which senior managers assess the implementation process to refine strategies and performance measures. Using performance statistics from the most recent period, managers identify flaws in strategies, obstacles to implementation efforts, critical changes in planning assumptions, and omissions in performance measures. Managers then develop refined strategies and measures to be implemented in the new year. The revised strategies and measures are then revisited during each subsequent annual gaming session to compare actual and expected performance.

In our earlier example, the regional system could review the employed primary care physicians' performance by periodically assessing actual productivity performance at each practice site against established targets. Gaming variables could include the number of visits by physician and practice site, referrals within the system, and changes in the market and environment. From this assessment, the management team could then refine physician incentive plans tied to practice productivity levels, or close sites, or decide to terminate practice agreements.

Anecdotal Reporting

Many of the measures that organizations use to gauge performance require substantial elapsed time or significant statistical data gathering before results can be judged. The time lag can be reduced by soliciting anecdotal reports on the strategy implementation efforts. Although not a substitute for rigorous statistical performance data, anecdotal information can be an early indicator of implementation results, until the more complete picture is available.

In our earlier example, the regional system could begin assessing the impact of its primary care strategy prior to the availability of complete market share data, which often lags by twelve to eighteen months. The system could analyze its own utilization levels of key volume indicators by residents of the targeted market to discern whether there appears to be an upward trend, either in absolute numbers or percentage. Even simpler would be an informal survey of the office staff of key physician specialists to ascertain how often their offices have been contacted for appointments by the primary care practitioners' offices.

Initiative Review

Organizations often develop more than one initiative to achieve strategic targets. These initiatives are usually tied to performance measures to gauge the level of success. Analyzing each initiative individually is an important feedback tool in assessing its impact on achieving the collective strategic objective.

For example, if increasing the number of patients seen in the primary care practices in outlying areas is a target in our previous example, a supporting initiative would be to ensure that any new patient calling for an initial appointment can be scheduled within three days. Evaluating the success of this well-defined initiative helps the organization understand its effectiveness.

Peer Review

Peer review is a traditional tool in all professional service industries to avoid groupthink and maintain strategic perspective. In most organizations, this mechanism is most effective if it occurs across departments or divisions. A small team of three to five managers from one division or department reviews another division or department's performance measures and strategic initiatives. The team then offers its independent feedback of the strategy and implementation process. This review should occur as often as is productive for each organization, typically annually or semiannually.

Hospital systems routinely employ peer review in leveraging the expertise of individual hospital management teams among the other system providers. For example, if one hospital team has excelled in productivity performance in its primary care physician practices, the team of managers would visit, evaluate, and make suggestions for improvements in this area to other hospitals within the system.

Limitations to Measures of Success

Performance measures are a key element of assessing the effectiveness of strategy implementation. However, they are only as credible as the data they reflect. Data accuracy and data intensity are common problem areas in performance measure assessments. Information systems must be evaluated in the course of the planning process to determine if current systems meet the requirements necessary to adequately measure organizational performance.

Conclusions

Many traditionally successful health care organizations have found that they are underequipped to implement strategic intent in the current dynamic environment. To be successful today, senior management must take an active and directive role in leading the transition. The CEO and the management team must define the vision, supply energy, focus roles and relationships for the organization, and serve as role models in the change process. Because the implementation path is changeable and uncertain, the organizational culture must encourage prudent risk taking and be flexible in implementation.

Lessons Learned

✓ Senior management must visibly lead the implementation of strategic intent. The CEO and management team must energize, explain, lead by example, listen sympathetically, take decisive action, and celebrate successes.

✓ Consensus means agreement, not unanimity. In a dynamic environment, organizations must seek common ground but not allow the pace of change to be dictated by the person least willing to change.

✓ Organizational culture must match the desired strategic intent. In a clash between strategic intent and culture, the latter prevails.

✓ Management must gain and maintain the support of key leaders on the board and among the medical staff for successful implementation. Physician leaders must be partners in the change process.

✓ The board must fully understand the potential capital and human costs of change, accept the risks associated with strategic intent, and be prepared to allocate or reallocate the resources needed to achieve agreed-upon objectives.

✓ Management must plan for short-term wins, regularly communicate progress, and be flexible in modifying action steps and personnel assignments to overcome obstacles.

✓ Senior management's leadership role is perhaps greatest in managing the human side of change and guiding the transition from the old ways to establishment of strategic intent.

✓ Health care organizations must develop structured organizational learning mechanisms if they are to capture hard-won lessons and build on both their mistakes and successes.

10

Summary and Conclusions

Marian C. Jennings

The tools and processes outlined in the previous chapters are meant to be practical approaches to enhancing health care strategic planning. Over the next decade, it is likely that biotechnology and information technology changes, societal expectations, demographic trends, and financial pressures will challenge the U.S. health care system in unprecedented ways. What is uncertain is the magnitude and timing of the pressures, and the exact forms they will take. These uncertainties would challenge any industry, but health care is different. Unlike much of the consumer products industry that drives the American economy, health care is in and of itself a necessary societal good.

The health care system is facing its greatest challenges simultaneously with increased demands from the so-called baby boom generation. Just as the need for a stable, vibrant health care system increases, the overall industry structure is showing stress fractures. The current system, where insurers, employers, providers, and consumers all are unhappy, is unstable and cannot continue. As has been true in all industries, the health care system will reestablish equilibrium, albeit in a new form and with structures different from today's. During the shakeout phase, there will continue to be an increasing separation between winning and losing organizations.

In this final chapter, we examine the traditional planning tools and processes that remain valid during the upcoming tumultuous period, identify where fundamental changes in techniques and processes are needed, and summarize a final set of lessons learned— often the hard way.

Certain Traditional Planning Processes Still Valid

In our experience, five traditional planning processes constitute a solid foundation for tomorrow's strategic setting processes:

1. Developing a common, objective understanding of the organization's starting position
2. Developing a clear and compelling vision for the future
3. Identifying clear, measurable objectives or targets
4. Committing to effective implementation processes, with clear-cut authorities and responsibilities identified
5. Integrating strategic and financial planning

The Market Assessment

First, strategic direction in an era of uncertainty must be built on an objective, thorough understanding of the health care environment, the organization's market, and its current positioning in that market. Nothing sounds more obvious than this. However, over the past decade, unlike their counterparts in corporate America, many hospitals and health systems have paid only lip service to this effort. When asked for their market assessments, organizations too often present either a set of generic, global health care trends, extracted from industry gurus and accepted as givens, or else mind-numbing reams of detailed data (market share by twenty-five zip code areas for thirteen service lines).

As described in Chapter Three, health care organizations need well-structured information that clearly highlights key trends, enhances understanding of the unknowns that are knowable, and identifies the major environmental risks or uncertainties facing the organization. The qualitative and quantitative information must be compiled objectively, facilitating a realistic assessment of organizational competencies, strengths, and weaknesses. Greater recognition of the increasingly sophisticated consumer must be built into the market assessment, using tools commonly employed in the corporate world, namely, structured focus groups and formal consumer market research.

Finally, the market assessment also should inform the organization of how well it has progressed against previously established goals and targets. For example, a regional health care system established a goal and related strategies in the mid-1990s to increase its presence and market share in seven outlying counties. As part of its 1999 market assessment, staff wanted to update the market share trends in these outlying counties. However, when senior management realized that these data would show no increases in market position, their immediate reaction was to exclude this trend information from the assessment since they did not want board members or physicians to lose confidence in the current planning effort. A more appropriate and productive approach would be to include the trend data, and use this portion of the market assessment to stimulate discussion of whether the former goal is still appropriate; if yes, which new approaches should be used and which obstacles to implementation still need to be overcome?

Clear, Compelling Vision Statement

A short, compelling statement of vision or strategic intent is the core of any strategic direction setting. A good vision statement is one that is memorable, compelling, and differentiating. In many organizations, the word *vision* has been overused and a new term should be coined to engender enthusiasm. Regardless of what it is called, a vision that imparts an easily communicated and understood picture of where the organization will be in three to five years should receive considerable time and attention during the strategy-setting process.

Tangible Measures of Success

The third traditional planning approach that is still valid is establishing tangible, quantifiable objectives or measures of success. Such tangible outcomes help to clarify the vision for all participants. Although many individuals who participate in the strategy-setting processes are conceptual thinkers, inevitably others think more concretely. For those who prefer concrete actions to ideas, setting clear objectives and targets greatly helps them understand the overall vision and strategy of the organization.

To be most useful in an era of uncertainty, the objectives and measures of success should be as specific and measurable as possible, with clear timetables for implementation. Establishing such specific targets can be challenging for those organizations whose past planning objectives have focused more on process than outcome. For example, one hospital traditionally used process-related terminology for its objectives ("Assess the feasibility of . . ."). Another was used to vague terminology ("Increase market share . . .") without articulating any specific targets.

The planning facilitator should demand that the organization be specific, even if this is an uncomfortable and time-consuming effort. Specific objectives and targets allow the organization to measure its progress in implementing its strategic intent and assist the organization in reevaluating how appropriate strategies are. For market-adapter organizations in particular, having in place specific targets is necessary to ensure the adaptability and flexibility implied by its preferred strategic intent.

Effective Implementation

Actions speak louder than words. Implementation has long been the hallmark of successful organizations of all types. As described in Chapter Nine, effective implementation in an era of uncertainty is harder to accomplish but more important than ever. Leaders, including board members, senior and midlevel managers and physicians, as well as associates, must commit themselves to focused action—while recognizing the possibility that their actions may not be sufficient to accomplish the desired results.

Integration of Strategic and Financial Planning

As the risks in the environment increase, so does the need to integrate strategic planning and financial planning efforts. Historically, most health care organizations have had access to capital when needed. Many organizations are facing a future in which their ability to borrow will be constrained, or they will be unwilling to assume the risks associated with additional debt. Therefore, the organization must make sure that it is allocating capital in a manner that supports its vision and strategic intent.

Traditional approaches to integrating strategic and financial planning are still valid. Typically, these include incorporating a financial capability analysis into the environmental assessment, developing baseline financial forecasts, identifying the capital and operating costs associated with strategy implementation, generating expected financial results and return on investment for the major strategic initiatives, and conducting sensitivity analyses to model the potential impacts of major environmental uncertainties.

Aspects of Traditional Approaches to Change or Abandon

Many of the traditional approaches to strategic planning are still appropriate in an era of uncertainty, but other approaches should be revamped, discarded, or augmented. Specifically, changes are needed in five areas.

First, formulate and use planning assumptions in new ways. Now, planning assumptions must address explicitly the uncertainties of the future environment. Planning assumptions should no longer articulate one expected future but instead should be organized and presented around the three major categories of uncertainty discussed in Chapter One: clear trends, unknowns that are knowable, and residual uncertainties. Special attention should be paid to the residual uncertainties that could have the greatest impact on the organization's ability to succeed. Implications of the planning assumptions should be clearly articulated and communicated; then goals and strategies should be connected back to these key assumptions.

Second, explicitly incorporate uncertainty and risk into the planning process. As described in detail in Chapter Five, health care organizations should use new tools for constructing their strategic plans. Specifically, in developing strategic intent, tools such as scenario planning, decision analysis, and game theory allow participants to address the uncertainties productively. Although these tools do not eliminate the uncertainties and risks associated with implementation, they do help organizations understand the nature of the risks they could be assuming, and assess the risk preference of the organization.

Third, shorten the planning cycle time frame. Planning in a dynamic, uncertain market implies a shortened strategic horizon, say, three years rather than five to ten years. However, certain long-term initiatives, such as improving the health of communities, require a longer perspective. Such initiatives should not be eliminated from the plan nor expected to yield results more quickly than is reasonable. Instead, the organization should recognize the increased risks associated with such long-term efforts; identify clear, short-term measures of success for the initial stages of their implementation; and develop contingency plans up front.

Fourth, identify clear indicators that the market is moving away from the expected or preferred direction. Such trigger points help an organization know when it is appropriate to reassess its strategic intent and strategies. An additional benefit of such trigger points is that by specifying the type of market changes that warrant concern, they keep the organization from endlessly reexamining its assumptions and strategic direction every time something changes in the environment.

As described in Chapter Seven, to be valuable, both trigger points and metrics must be clearly stated and easily and routinely monitored. An example of a clear trigger point is "Community Hospital announces a merger with University Hospital." Indicators that are too vague ("The market continues to consolidate") are open to too much interpretation or unwarranted action. For example, a competitor's acquisition of an ambulatory care center might be of little consequence but fall within the definition of the latter sort of trigger point. Similarly, metrics are not useful if they require extensive research or information that is difficult to gather, such as "Our quality of clinical care is consistently in the top quartile of hospitals in our region."

Fifth, reduce the organization's exposure to risks in the implementation phase by incorporating measures of success and targets, and by developing contingency plans at the outset for the riskiest strategies. The measures of success and targets afford clear, short-term, tangible expectations of outcomes. Failure to achieve a target should trigger reexamination of its causes. Was implementation slow or incomplete? If so, focus additional management time and resources on enhancing planned efforts. Did the actions succeed but fail to generate the desired outcome? If so, reexamine the strategic initiatives and identify new, potentially more effective initiatives. Has there been a market shift that means it is time to reexamine strategies or even goals? If so, honestly reassess overall progress in implementing strategic intent and make any necessary changes.

Contingency plans should be developed for those strategic initiatives that carry special risks. Contingency planning is particularly important when an initiative (1) is capital-intensive, (2) is expected to generate most of its financial return more than three years out, or (3) involves a change in the organization's cost structure that would be difficult to reverse (such as a policy decision about staffing that increases employee wages and benefits). There also are nonfinancial risks that can require contingency planning; two examples are an initiative that risks changing a hospital's image in the community from that of a good citizen to that of a fierce competitor, and an initiative that closely aligns selected physicians with a system but risks alienating other medical staff members. Contingency plans should not be developed as doomsday scenarios but rather as legitimate vehicles to reduce the organization's risk exposure.

Lessons Learned

Each chapter has presented its related key lessons, which are not reiterated here. Instead, this set of lessons learned reflects observations gathered in working with numerous health care organizations of all sizes across the country, each facing its own environment and challenges, all starting from different competitive positions, and demonstrating quite diverse cultures.

✓ Lesson one: strategic planning can be a transformational process for the organization. Hospitals and health care systems are in the midst of a fundamental industrywide restructuring effort. This restructuring can create great organizational anxiety, in which concern and fear about the future can immobilize and demoralize senior leadership, physicians, managers and directors, and employees alike. Explicit consideration of the uncertainties of the future can help to build the organization's sense of selecting and charting its own future course, albeit in turbulent waters.

✓ Lesson two: to be effective, strategic planning must be led from the top. A key role of the CEO is to develop a vision and direction for the organization he or she leads. In our experience, participative planning processes in today's environment yield results only with clear CEO commitment to the process, outcomes, and implementation. In addition, the board must be willing to acknowledge the uncertainties of the future environment and not require unmitigated successes.

✓ Lesson three: me-too strategies rarely work. Many organizations take comfort in adopting the same strategies as those of their market competitors. However, strategy implies something unique.

Implementing other organizations' strategies fails to account for important differences among organizations, such as core ideology and culture, as well as in an organization's starting competitive advantages and vulnerabilities.

✓ Lesson four: culture and strategy are inextricably linked. An organization must assess its culture honestly, early in the planning process, and recognize the power of that culture to support or inhibit its strategic direction. If the preferred strategic intent does not fit with the current culture, specific strategies to transform the culture must be incorporated into the strategic plan or else the strategic intent must be modified. Otherwise, the organization faces the likelihood of failing in plan implementation, causing frustration and lessening support for future planning efforts.

✓ Lesson five: although many hospitals and health systems perceive themselves to be market adapters, they lack the agility and flexibility required in this role. Often, the market adapter role is selected by default. The organization recognizes that it is too risk-averse to be a true market enactor, but it wants to be more than a market survivor. Therefore, it articulates a market-adapter intent. If your organization's strategic intent is to be an adapter, ask yourselves two questions: "Have we demonstrated our willingness to exit a market or a service?" "In what recent decision have we demonstrated our flexibility or agility?" If the answers yield few or no examples, it is essential that your organization begin to experiment with adapterlike behaviors to build this core competence.

✓ Lesson six: beware of lowest-common-denominator strategies. In periods of uncertainty, the desire to have a unified team may increase. However, each participant has an individual tolerance for risk. Attempts to reach consensus, even in its true meaning of general agreement, may result in selecting strategies that are perceived to be less risky, such as status quo or incremental approaches. Over time, a series of these presumably less risky, incremental strategies may stall organizational momentum and substantially increase organizational risk. To avoid this, at least one member of the management team should be appointed the devil's advocate, charged with challenging the group whenever its thinking moves toward weak, diluted strategies.

✓ Lesson seven: successful implementation no longer guarantees the desired results. One of the most painful lessons of planning in an era of uncertainty is that even the best and the brightest managers no longer can guarantee good results. As discussed throughout this book, a dynamic market requires an organization to constantly and objectively evaluate the successes or failures of strategies; to discriminate between appropriately "staying the course" and stubbornly refusing to reexamine strategies; and to willingly abandon a strategy when required.

✓ Lesson eight: a brilliant strategy without the needed financial resources to carry it out is no strategy at all. Strategic planning is essentially a resource allocation process. All too often, organizations divorce their strategic intent from the capital budgeting process, underestimate the magnitude of the investment required to implement strategic intent, or expect a return within an unrealistically short time frame. To ensure that adequate resources to implement strategy are available, organizations should continue to build, or at least maintain, their cash and investments. Though this can be difficult given the financial pressures facing the industry, we believe that maintaining this financial flexibility is critical to ensuring that today's health care organization is vibrant at the end of the next decade.

Conclusion

The approaches, techniques, and lessons learned described in this chapter and throughout this book give health care leaders a practical toolkit with which to carry out strategic planning differently and more effectively in a new and unfamiliar health care environment. Our hope is that this book has stimulated you to recommitment to formal strategic planning processes for your organization. Now more than ever, health care organizations need systematic planning processes that lead to a limited set of focused strategic initiatives. As never before, organizations need the insight to consciously choose a specific strategic intent to the exclusion of others, and the courage to transform themselves in the planning process.

We hope that this book has resonated with board members, chief executive officers, vice presidents or directors of strategic planning, chief financial officers, and others involved in the strategic planning process. We hope that you have gained insight into the art and the science of strategic planning and that you have been inspired to challenge conventional approaches and thinking in your own organization.

Glossary of Terms

Balanced scorecard Planning tool that monitors financial performance while simultaneously measuring progress in improving market position, meeting owner and customer needs, and enhancing internal business processes.

Benchmarking Valuable tool in the environmental assessment process, allowing an organization to compare its performance in key areas to those of competitors or industry peers.

Big bets High-risk strategies requiring considerable investment of resources with the potential for great payoffs (or losses).

Clear trends Trends that are readily identifiable, such as demographics, continued pressure on prices, declining use rates, and introduction of new technologies.

Core ideology Core ideology captures an organization's core purpose and values. Core ideology, vision, and market stance combine to form strategic intent.

Core purpose A component of core ideology describing an organization's reason for being, generally captured in its mission statement.

Core values A component of core ideology describing the intrinsic beliefs that the organization values above all others and that characterize the best efforts of the company throughout changing market conditions.

Dashboard of key indicators An assessment device supplementing traditional financial measures with criteria that examine an organization's performance on nonfinancial indicators critical to the success of strategic initiatives.

Data   Factual information (for example, statistics) used as the basis for assessment or discussion.

Decision analysis   Decision-making process whereby an alternative is selected from two or more exclusive courses of action.

Delphi forecasting   A method used to elicit the opinions of experts through a series of repeated questions, while avoiding the potential biases of face-to-face panel discussions.

Environmental assessment   A thorough review of the internal and external conditions in which an organization operates. Also referred to as a situation audit.

Financial capability   The amount of capital an organization can raise and invest at an acceptable level of risk.

Game theory   The branch of social science that studies strategic thinking and decision making.

Goals   Desired end results toward which effort is directed.

Information   The communication of knowledge.

Issues questionnaire   A written survey designed to elicit input regarding individuals' expectations for the future.

Market adapter   A form of strategic intent in which organizations adopt strategies tailored to their best guesses about the direction of the market, while keeping their options open.

Market enactor   A form of strategic intent in which an organization approaches market uncertainty by trying to change factors in its environment to its strategic advantage.

Market stance   A component of strategic intent that describes how the organization chooses to go about realizing its vision, based on its risk preference, corporate culture, current strategic position, and financial capacity.

Market survivor   A form of strategic intent in which an organization waits until the environment becomes certain and focuses on incremental, operational, no-regrets moves rather than strategies.

Measures of success   Collectively, a benchmark to monitor an organization's progress toward successful implementation of its strategic intent and specific strategies and test the validity of an organization's planning assumptions.

Metric   Internal indicator that monitors the organization's short-term performance related to the implementation of its long-term strategies.

Mission   A statement describing an organization's core purpose or reason for being.

New path   Tool that can help an organization define its market stance. The "game board" is a visual representation of the various dimensions of the organization's services and how it delivers those services. For each dimension, there are alternative strategies that could be pursued.

No-regrets moves   Operational initiatives such as improving infra-structure and customer focus, reducing costs, and improving quality. These incremental, operational moves are important to the ongoing success of any organization, but they are not substitutes for strategy.

Planning assumptions   "Best guesses" about the future that specify expectations regarding the external environment and implications for organizational success.

Residual uncertainty   Remaining unknowns after clear trends and unknowns that are knowable are identified; uncertainties that are not made clear through further research effort.

Scenario planning   Planning technique that challenges traditional thinking through alternative futures that identify strategic options and risks.

Stakeholders   Those having a vested interest in a common enterprise.

Strategic information   The combination of data in a format that communicates information useful to the strategic planning process.

Strategic intent   The combination of core ideology, vision, and market stance, defining an organization's corporate identity and pre-ferred future direction.

Strategies   Carefully designed plans for deploying resources to attain a favorable position.

Triggers; trigger points   Market indicators used to determine whether the organization's planning assumptions still hold true for strategy implementation.

Unknowns that are knowable   Type of uncertainty that is neither a clear trend nor entirely unpredictable; uncertainties that can become clearer with additional research. Educated guesses are effective in making predictions with some degree of confidence.

Vision   A component of strategic intent in the form of a descriptive statement about where the organization wants to position itself for the future.

References

Advocate Health Care. 1998. http://www.advocatehealth.com/about/mvphil.html.

"Atlanta MCOs Collaborating on Guidelines with Competitors." *Managed Care Outlook*, Apr. 2, 1999, p. 3.

Bell, C. W. "Staying Fit: Providers Would Do Best to Leverage Giving, Plan for Worst." *Modern Healthcare*, June 7, 1999, p. 32.

Bezold, C. "Five Futures." *Healthcare Forum Journal*, May/June 1992, pp. 29–42.

Brandenburger, A. M., and Nalebuff, B. J. "The Right Game: Use Game Theory to Shape Strategy." *Harvard Business Review*, July–Aug. 1995, pp. 57–71.

Brandenburger, A. M., and Nalebuff, B. J. *Co-opetition*. New York: Bantam Doubleday, 1996.

Brasel, K. J., M.D., and Weigelt, J., M.D. "Decision Analysis: Balancing Quality and Cost." *Infection Control and Hospital Epidemiology*, Feb. 1997, *18*, 146–148.

Bridges, W. *Managing Transitions: Making the Most of Change*. Reading, Mass.: Addison-Wesley, 1991.

Campbell, A., and Alexander, M. "What's Wrong with Strategy?" *Harvard Business Review*, Nov.–Dec. 1997, *74*, 42.

Catholic Health East. 1999. http://www.chenet.org/core.html.

"Chicago's Northwestern Healthcare System Unravels." *Healthcare Financial Management*, Aug. 1999, *53*, 18.

Coile, R. C. *Beyond 2000: Health Care Trends in the New Millennium*. Chicago: Society for Healthcare Strategy and Market Development, American Hospital Association, 1999.

Collins, J. C., and Porras, J. I. "Building Your Company's Vision." *Harvard Business Review*, Sept.–Oct. 1996, p. 66.

"A Comprehensive Review of Hospital Finances in the Aftermath of the Balanced Budget Act of 1997." Washington, D.C.: Ernst and Young, LLP, and HCIA, Inc., Mar. 1999.

Courtney, H., Kirkland, J., and Viguerie, P. "Strategy Under Uncertainty." *Harvard Business Review*, Nov.–Dec. 1997, *77*, 68.

Courtney, H., Kirkland, J., and Viguerie, P. *Harvard Business Review on Managing Uncertainty*. Boston: Harvard Business School Press, 1999.

Davis, M. D. *Game Theory: A Nontechnical Introduction*. Mineola, N.Y.: Dover, 1983.

Dawes, R. M. *Rational Choice in an Uncertain World*. Orlando: Harcourt Brace, 1988.

Dixit, A. K., and Nalebuff, B. J. *Thinking Strategically*. New York: Norton, 1991.

Duck, J. D. *Managing Change: The Art of Balancing*. (Harvard Business Review on Change.) Boston: Harvard Business School Press, 1998. (Originally published in *Harvard Business Review*, Nov.–Dec. 1993)

Feder, B. J. "Plotting Corporate Futures: Outlining What Could Go Wrong." *New York Times*, June 24, 1999.

FedEx. (n.d.) http://www.fedex.com.

"For the Record: Healthcare Giving Jumps." *Modern Healthcare*, May 31, 1999a, p. 17.

"For the Record: Long-Term Care Company Files Chapter 11." *Modern Healthcare*, June 28, 1999b, p. 16.

Gilkey, R. W. (ed.). *The 21st Century Health Care Leader*. San Francisco: Jossey-Bass, 1999.

Goldstein, L. "Moody's Foresees Increase in Number of Not-for-Profit Healthcare Speculative-Grade Ratings over the Intermediate Term." *Moody's Investors Service*, July 14, 1999.

Goleman, D. *Emotional Intelligence*. New York: Bantam Books, 1997.

Goodman, T. *The Forbes Book of Business Quotations*. New York: Black Dog and Leventhal, 1997.

Goss, T., Pascale, R., and Athos, A. *The Reinvention Roller Coaster*. (Harvard Business Review on Change.) Boston: Harvard Business School Press, 1998. (Originally published in *Harvard Business Review*, Nov.–Dec. 1993)

Governance Institute. "The Meaning of Columbia/HCA: Understanding Their Role as an Agent of Change." (Governance One Hundred.) La Jolla, Calif.: Governance Institute, 1996.

Hensley, S. "AHERF Files for Chapter 11." *Modern Healthcare*, July 27, 1998, pp. 2–3.

"Highlights of Clinton Medicare Plan." *New York Times*, June 29, 1999.
    [Reprinted on http://www.nytimes.com]

Hofer, C. W., and Schendel, D. *Strategy Formulation: Analytical Concepts.*
    St. Paul: West, 1978.

Hudson, T. "Choose Your Tomorrow." *Hospitals and Health Networks*, Aug. 20,
    1995, pp. 38–40.

Hudson, T., Haugh, R., and Serb, C. "Off Target." *Hospitals and Health Networks*,
    Jan. 1999, *73*, 35.

Ingalls, L. "Scenario Planning for Effective Facilities Decisions." 1999.
    www.fmdata.com/fmdm/issues/9904/MDACC/.

Jaklevic, M. C. "Docs Hit by FPA Filing." *Modern Healthcare*, July 27, 1998, p. 6.

Jennings, M. C. (ed.). *Financially-Driven Strategic Planning.* Frederick, Md.:
    Aspen, 1998.

Kaplan, R. S., and Norton, D. P. *Translating Strategy into Action: The Balanced
    Scorecard.* Boston: Harvard Business School Press, 1996a.

Kaplan, R., and Norton, D. "Using the Balanced Scorecard as a Strategic Man-
    agement System." *Harvard Business Review*, Jan.–Feb. 1996b, p. 75.

Kichheimer, B. "Fallout from Nowhere." *Modern Healthcare*, Apr. 5, 1999, p. 36.

Kleinmuntz, D. N., Kleinmuntz, C. E., Stephen, R. G., and Nordlund, D. S.
    "Measuring and Managing Risk Improves Strategic Financial Planning."
    Healthcare Financial Management, June 1999, *53*, 51.

Kolb, D. S. (ed.). *Assessing Organizational Readiness for Capitation.* Chicago:
    American Hospital Publishing, 1996.

Kotter, J. P. "Leading Change: Why Transformation Efforts Fail." *Harvard Busi-
    ness Review*, Mar.–Apr. 1995, p. 63.

Lilford, J., Parker, S. G., Braunholtz, D. A., and Chard, J. "Decision Analysis
    and the Implementation of Research Findings." *BMJ*, Aug. 8, 1998, *317*,
    405–409.

MacCracken, L. *Market-Driven Strategy: An Executive Guide to Health Care's
    Integrated Environment.* Chicago: American Hospital Publishing, 1998.

McCafferty, J. "Critical Condition: Why Health Care CFOs Have the Toughest
    Finance Jobs in America." *CFO*, Jan. 1999, pp. 63–71.

McCarthy, L. "New Jersey Officials Seek to Liquidate HIP Health Plans; Viable
    Alternatives Lacking." *BNA's Managed Care Reporter*, Feb. 1999, *7*, 159.

McGill, M. E., and Slocum, J. W., Jr. *The Smarter Organization: How to Build a Busi-
    ness That Learns and Adapts to Marketplace Needs.* New York: Wiley, 1994.

McGrath, G., and MacMillan, I. C. "Discovery-Driven Planning." *Harvard Busi-
    ness Review*, July–Aug. 1995, *73*, 45–46.

McWhinney, W., and others. *Creating Paths of Change: Revitalization, Renaissance, and Work*. Venice, Calif.: Enthusion, 1993.

Meyer, H. "Focused Factories: Are You Ready for the Competition?" *Hospitals and Health Networks*, Apr. 5, 1998, 72, 24.

Miles, R. E., and Snow, C. C. *Organizational Strategy, Structure and Process*. New York: McGraw-Hill, 1978.

Mintzberg, H. "The Rise and Fall of Strategic Planning." *Harvard Business Review*, Jan.–Feb. 1994, 72, 108.

Moore, J. D., Jr. "Chasm Grows Between Rich and Poor." *Modern Healthcare*, June 7, 1999a, p. 34.

Moore, J. D., Jr. "HMOs Cause Systems' Rating Hits." *Modern Healthcare*, Feb. 22, 1999b, p. 2.

"News at Deadline: Home Health Corporation of America." *Modern Healthcare*, Feb. 22, 1999, p. 4.

Peters, J. "Why Medical Groups Fail: There's Truth in the Numbers." *Health Care Strategic Management*, Aug. 1999, 17, 18.

Porter, M. E. "Competitive Advantage: Creating and Sustaining Superior Performance." New York: Free Press, 1985.

Porter, M. E. "What Is Strategy?" *Harvard Business Review*, Nov.–Dec. 1996, 74, 70.

Robinet, J.-E. "Competition: For Better or Worse." *Pittsburgh Business Times*, Apr. 12, 1999.

Shoemaker, P.J.H. "Scenario Planning: A Tool for Strategic Thinking." *Sloan Management Review*, Winter 1995, p. 26. (Originally published in Cerf, C., and Navasky, V. *The Experts Speak*. New York: Pantheon, 1984)

Starr, P. *The Social Transformation of American Medicine*. Boston: Basic Books, 1982.

"Strategic Planning Committees." (Fact brief.) Advisory Board Co., Jan. 1997, p. 1.

Sull, D. N. "Why Good Companies Go Bad." *Harvard Business Review*, July–Aug. 1999, pp. 44–45.

Sullivan, G. R. *Hope Is Not a Method*. New York: Random House, 1996.

"Think Tank Predicts Nuclear War Between India and Pakistan." Pakistan News Service, 1999. http://www.paknews.org.

Toner, R. "A Last, Modest Try at Health Reform." *New York Times*, July 4, 1999. [Reprinted on http://www.nytimes.com]

Tufte, E. *The Visual Display of Quantitative Information*. Cheshire, Conn.: Graphics Press, 1983.

U.S. Postal Service. (n.d.) http://www.usps.com.

Voelker, R. "Emergency Departments Open New Doors to Technology, Patient
    Service." *Journal of the American Medical Association*, Aug. 25, 1999, *282*,
    719–720.
Webber, J. P., and Peters, J. P. *Strategic Thinking: A New Frontier for Hospital
    Management.* Chicago: American Hospital Publishing, 1983.
Wernerfelt, B., and Karnani, A. "Competitive Strategy Under Uncertainty."
    Strategic Management Journal, Feb. 1987, *8*, 189.
Williams, J. R. *Renewable Advantage: Crafting Strategy Through Economic Time.*
    New York: Free Press, 1998.

Suggested Reading

Aaker, D. A. *Strategic Market Management.* (4th ed.) New York: Wiley, 1995.

American Management Association. "Encouraging a Risk Taking Culture." *Supervisory Management,* Aug. 1994, 8, 1–2.

Backer, T. E. "Managing the Human Side of Change in the VA's Transformation." *Hospital and Health Services Administration,* Fall 1997, 3, 433–459.

Beer, M., Eisenstat, F. A., and Spector, B. "Why Change Programs Don't Produce Change." *Harvard Business Review,* Nov.–Dec. 1990, pp. 158–166.

Chow, C. W., Ganulin, D., Haddad, K., and Williamson, J. "The Balanced Scorecard: A Potent Tool for Energizing and Focusing Healthcare Organization Management." *Journal of Healthcare Management,* May–June 1998, 3, 263–280.

Collins, J. C., and Porras, J. I. *Built to Last.* New York: HarperCollins, 1997.

Collins, J. "Turning Goals into Results: The Power of Catalytic Mechanisms." *Harvard Business Review,* July–Aug. 1999, pp. 71–82.

Eccles, R. G. "The Performance Measurement Manifesto." *Harvard Business Review* reprint collection, Jan.–Feb. 1991, pp. 56–62.

Gilkey, R. W., and Lieberman, G. R. "Blending Health Care Organizations." In R. W. Gilkey (ed.), *The 21st Century Health Care Leader.* San Francisco: Jossey-Bass, 1999.

Hammond, J. S., Keeney, R. L., and Raiffa, H. *Smart Choices: A Practical Guide to Making Better Decisions.* Boston: Harvard Business School Press, 1999.

Harvard Business Review on Managing Uncertainty. Boston: Harvard Business School Press, 1999.

Hodge, B. J., Anthony, W. P., and Gales, L. M. *Organization Theory: A Strategic Approach.* (5th ed.) Upper Saddle River, N.J.: Prentice Hall, 1996.

Ingersoll, J. E., and Ross, S. A. "Waiting to Invest: Investment and Uncertainty." *Journal of Business*, 1992, *1*, 1–29.

Kaplan, R. S., and Norton, D. P. "The Balanced Scorecard: Measures That Drive Performance." *Harvard Business Review* reprint collection, Jan.–Feb. 1992, pp. 64–72.

Kester, W. C. "Today's Options for Tomorrow's Growth." *Harvard Business Review*, Mar.–Apr. 1984, *2*, 153–160.

Kotter, J. P. "Leading Change: Why Transformation Efforts Fail." *Harvard Business Review*, Mar.–Apr. 1995, pp. 59–67.

Rosner, B. "How Do I Support Risk-Taking?" *Workforce*, Sept. 1998, *9*, 20–21.

Ryan, J. B., and Ward, M. E. "Capital Management." *Topics in Health Care Financing*, 1992, *19*(1).

Ryan, J. B., Ward, M. E., and Kolb, D. S. "Capital Management Balances Charitable, Financial Goals." *Healthcare Financial Management*, Mar. 1990, *3*, 32–40.

Schwartz, P. *The Art of the Long View*. New York: Doubleday, 1996.

Smith, M. "The Development of an Innovative Culture (Strategies to Encourage an Innovative Risk-Taking Culture)." *Management Accounting*, 1998, *76*(2), 22–23.

Starr, P. *The Social Transformation of American Medicine*. Boston: Basic Books, 1982.

Steiner, G. *Strategic Planning: A Step-by-Step Guide*. New York: Simon & Schuster, 1997.

Thompson, A. A., Jr., and Strickland, A. J., III. *Strategy Formulation and Implementation*. Boston: Irwin, 1992.

Tichy, N. M. *The Leadership Engine: How Winning Companies Build Leaders at Every Level*. New York: HarperCollins, 1997.

Tufte, E. R. *Envisioning Information*. Cheshire, Conn.: Graphics Press, 1990.

Tufte, E. R. *Visual Explanations: Images and Quantities, Evidence and Narrative*. Cheshire, Conn.: Graphics Press, 1997.

"Where in the World Are the Ambulatory Benchmarking Data?" *Healthcare Benchmarks: The Newsletter of Best Practices*, Sept. 1998, *9*, 133–137.

Index